THE
complete
MAN

THE
complete
MAN

EDITED BY SUE SEDDON

WARD LOCK LIMITED · LONDON

© Ward Lock Limited 1987

First published in Great Britain in 1987
by Ward Lock Limited, 8 Clifford Street
London W1X 1RB, an Egmont Company

Designed by Hugh Schermuly

Jacket photographs: *front:* British Van Heusen;
back: Ann Taylor

Text filmset/set in Century Old Style 10/11 pt
by Multiplex Techniques Ltd.

Printed and bound in Italy by
Canale

British Library Cataloguing in Publication Data

Seddon, Sue (ed.)
  The complete man.
  1. Grooming for men
  I. Title
  646.7'2   RA777.8

ISBN 0-7063-6601-8

contents

hair

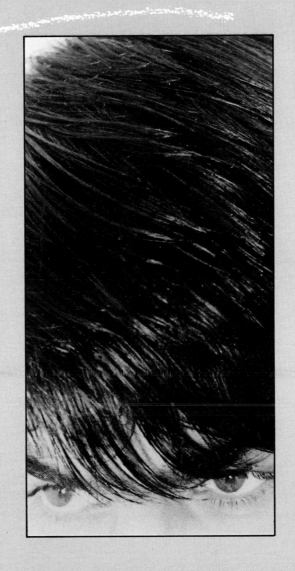

*B*arnet fair

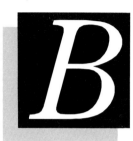

Every aspect of your life says something about the person within. The car you drive, the sports you play, the books you read and the clothes you wear all speak volumes about your lifestyle and personality. Yet hair is the one part of your appearance that gets used, abused and often downright neglected despite the fact that, properly cared for, it is capable of boosting your confidence and polishing your appearance to perfection.

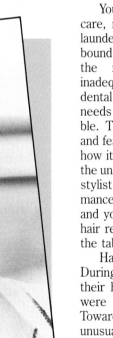

You clean a treasured vehicle with loving care, make sure your finest shirts are crisply laundered and cherish your favourite leather bound volumes for life. Hair gets yanked from the roots by cheap brushes, washed inadequately and haircuts are dealt with like dental appointments – a necessary chore that needs to be dispensed with as briskly as possible. The main reasons for this are ignorance and fear. Ignorance of what hair actually is and how it can look if handled properly and fear of the unknown: how to find a good salon, a helpful stylist and fear of actually demanding performance from your hair. Conquer these handicaps and you are well on your way to making your hair reflect the man, and in doing so, painting the tableau you want people to see.

Haircare is not just a woman's prerogative. During Elizabethan times men liked to wave their hair, sporting a love-lock or two which were sometimes tied with bright ribbons. Towards the end of the 18th century it was not unusual for a fashionable English gentleman to make the arrangement of his hair the main business of the day. Followers of Beau Brummel would often pass the morning selecting ribbons for their hair! You often admire a woman for her crowning glory, but the same applies in reverse. Female fans have fought for a strand of their pop idol's locks. Even if you are not blessed with a flowing mane, you can still make it look appealing. Telly Savalas shaved his head and became a hearthrob overnight.

Just as Buddhist monks shave their heads and Sikhs never cut their hair, it should make a statement about the man it adorns. "You can tell a great deal about a man from the way he wears his hair," says Joshua Galvin, eminent London hairdresser and salon owner. "Punks, teddy boys, hippies and skinheads wear their hair almost as part of their uniform, Yuppy, Sloaney types wear more conventional flat, parted styles and businessmen will always prefer neat, short haircuts."

It isn't necessary to preen your hair as much as the Regency bucks and dandies but at least take responsibility for it yourself. Look at the shampoo you use, does it really enhance your hair or is it left feeling lanky and heavy? Do you feel totally confident that your hairdresser or barber knows what you want? Do you tell him or her how you would like your hair to look or have you even mentioned any hair problems? "Men have no interest in buying products of their own volition," confirms Leslie Spears, chairman of 365 Day Hairdressing, an organization which helps hundreds of hairdressers make the most of their businesses. "The latent desire to care for hair is there, but it needs prodding. A man needs an icebreaker, something he can latch onto, to ignite an interest in his hair, whether it be a new stylist, a product, or a method of drying hair."

There's nothing new in making your hair your crowning glory and it's certainly nothing to be ashamed of or embarrassed by. Wealthy Elizabethan males made sure they obtained the fullest attention from their hairdresser by lodging over barbers shops in Fleet Street and The Strand when they visited London. Neither is it a sin to wear your hair long. The large and flamboyant full-bottomed wig popular amongst men of the 17th century had gone out of fashion by about 1720 but old men and professionals still insisted on wearing it for a further 20 years. Hair is a wonderful, delicate, sensual fibre. Treat it with respect, even if it isn't abundant, and it will pay dividends.

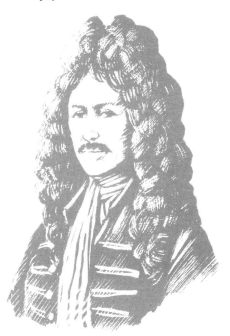

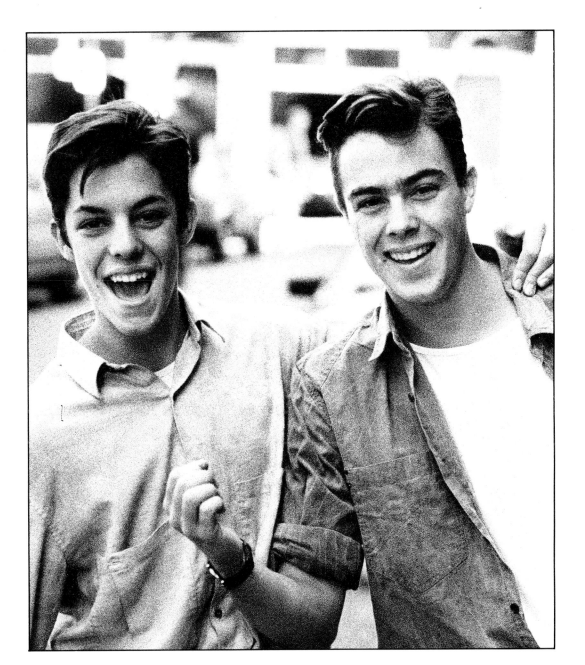

*H*air there and everywhere

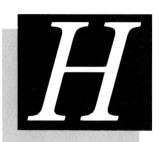

Hair is, in a way, a small miracle. There are between 80,000 and 150,000 hairs on a head and each one can be stronger than a copper wire of the same diameter. It protects, insulates, and identifies the owner and it can make or break your appearance. Lack of it has been known to drive strong men to drink or to the psychiatrist, while an abundant mane turns heads, stops hearts and, in the case of some models, leads to a fortune.

There are many myths in hair folklore, but it is not a myth that the hair you see on your head is dead. But that doesn't mean that it can be abused because the way in which you treat your hair makes a vital difference to the way it looks.

*W*HAT'S IN A HAIR?

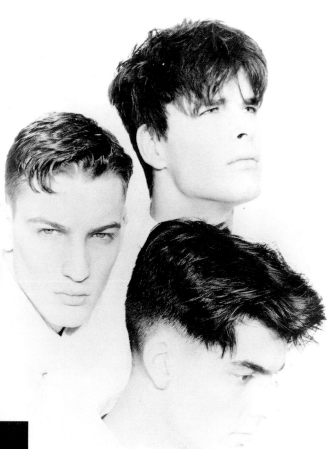

If those mis-used, much abused fibres on your head are to become its crowning glory it's important to know what hair is and how it grows. Each hair is clearly structured for growth, protection and colour. The hair shaft has three layers. The outer protective layer, or cuticle, acts rather like a good suit of armour. It is made up of overlapping transparent scales of strong protein or keratin. The scales open out when the hair is wet and close when it is dry. If your hair seems to be exuding good health it is because the cuticles are laying flat and reflecting the light, giving the hair a healthy sheen. If your hair is lack-lustre the scales may be damaged and unable to lie flat or reflect light so hair looks dull and out of sorts.

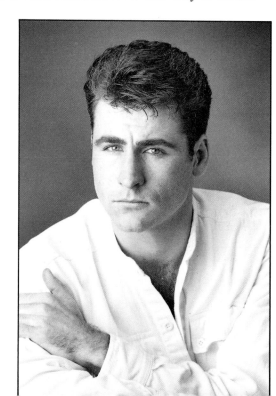

COLOUR CARRIERS

The cortex is the layer of the hair shaft that forms the main bulk of the hair. It contains cells that bond together to give stretch and strength to each hair. When all the bonds inside the hair are intact they are strong. As bonds break they become weaker, or sensitized.

The cortex also houses melanin, the pigment that determines the colour of hair. Blondes have small amounts of melanin. Brunettes have a combination of melanin and red pigment granules. Redheads have little melanin and lots of red pigment. When melanin cannot be made hair turns grey. The central core of hair is called the medulla and forms the thickness of each hair shaft. It is often missing in fine hair.

> *Hair in poor condition will break three times more quickly than hair in good condition.*
>
> *Hair in good condition is able to stretch to one third of its original length when wet and return when dry. Because the bonds are intact the hair will be bouncy and retain shape and movement. Hair in poor condition will stretch one third of its original length when wet but because of its weakened state, caused by broken bonds, it will not return when dry and loses shape quickly.*

A HAIR'S BREADTH

The thickness of hair can create colourful optical illusions. Blonde heads of hair appear the least abundant because this colour is the finest in diameter but blondes actually have the greatest number of hairs on their heads. Red hair is the thickest in diameter. Redheads often appear to have most hair but in fact they have fewer hairs per square inch than blondes. It is the coarseness of each red hair that creates the illusion of a very thick mane of hair.

Average amount of hair according to sex and hair colour		
	Female	Male
Natural Brown/ Black	130,000	100,000
Natural Blonde	150,000	130,000
Natural Red	80,000	80,000

HAIRY, HAIRY, HOW DOES YOUR THICK MANE GROW?

Hair starts life deep in the skin of the scalp, or the epidermis. The epidermis is fed by the dermis where follicles are found. Follicles have a rich supply of blood cells. The blood stimulates a clump of cells at the base of the follicle and they produce hair cells which grow, harden and die, becoming the hair shaft. The angle at which the follicle approaches the skin affects the shape of hair. Straight hair is the result of the follicle sitting vertically in the scalp. If it is bent or curved, curly hair is the result. Afro hair is elliptical, resulting in a mane of curls.

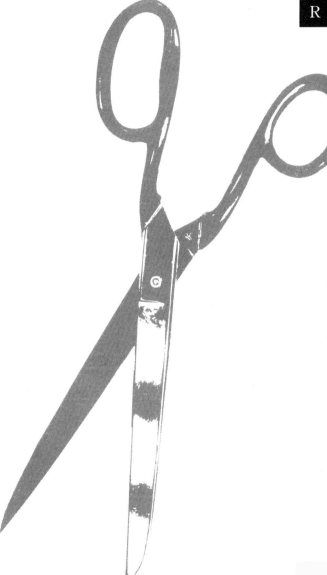

GROWTH RATE

Hair has three cycles of growth, the anagen, catagen and telogen phases. In the anagen phase the hair bulb stretches itself out into the follicle where it meets with keratin which seals and protects it. The duration of this stage determines how long hair will grow. Scalp hair grows at about half an inch per month. It usually lasts for between two and seven years but periods of 25 years have been recorded. Hair growth slows during the catagen stage and keratinization does not take place. Finally hair enters the telogen stage where it rests for between three or four months until the whole cycle begins again. During this stage hair is easily removed by washing and brushing.

NATURAL LUBRICATION

Each hair follicle has a sebaceous gland which produces sebum, the hair's natural lubricant. Sebum oils the hair shaft and skin and keeps them supple and smooth. When sebaceous glands become over active they produce too much sebum and the hair becomes greasy. When they aren't active enough there is too little sebum and the hair is dry.

DIET RIGHT

Treat your hair as you would the most delicate silk shirt, with kindness and consideration. There are many outside elements – sun, wind, sea and chemical treatments – all working together adversely to affect your hair. Help combat these enemies by taking a long hard look at your diet and lifestyle. Just as you wouldn't dream of washing that shirt in harsh detergent, neither should you feed your body

rubbish. Your external appearance is a reflection of what goes on inside your body. If you eat only faddy foods or lack essential vitamins and lead a continuously stressful life, don't expect a gleaming, bountiful head of hair in return.

> *Under normal conditions 85 to 95 per cent of coarse scalp hairs are in the anagen stage; one per cent in the catagen; and from four to fourteen per cent in the telogen stage. Nearly all of the tiny hairs on the scalp are in the telogen stage and on average, humans lose between 50 and 75 hairs per day.*

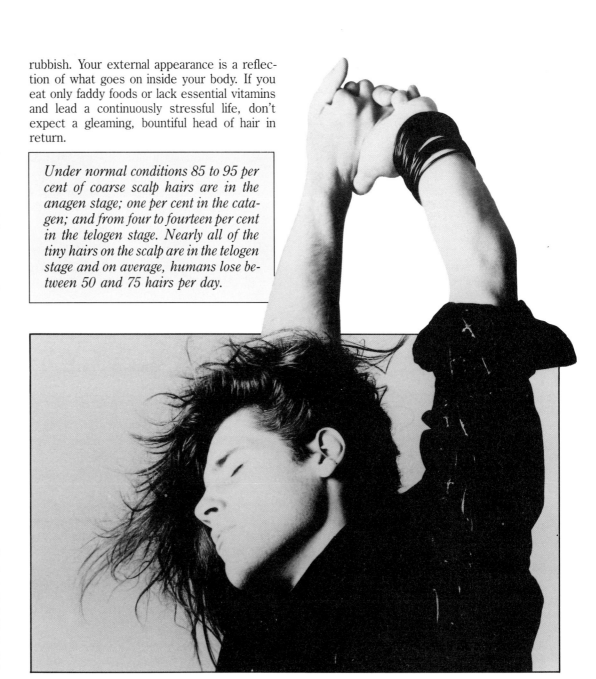

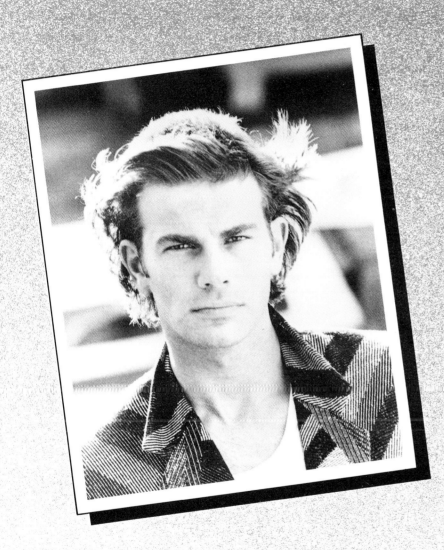

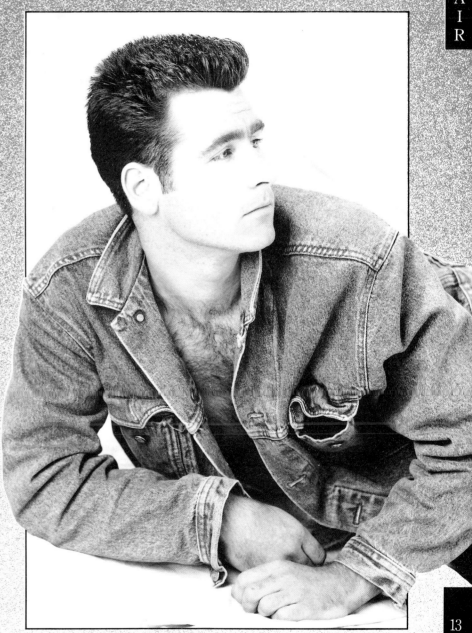

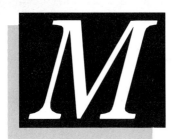aking headway

Hair can often appear to be much more of a problem than an asset and it is true that from time to time there are hiccups in its growth, health and manageability. Understanding something of the way it grows, and how you feed and nurture it, should help to conquer these problems. Unfortunately there are outside elements, many of them self-inflicted, which can still interfere with your hair's well-being. Knowing what the common problems are and how to combat them is vital to a healthy head of hair. Some of the cruellest conditions you subject your hair to are part and parcel of a normal day. But become aware of them and soften the blow by taking protective measures or cutting down on exposure time.

Man-made conditions can affect hair just as adversely as nature's. Central heating dries the air and leaves hair parched. Put back essential moisture into the atmosphere by either using humidifiers or placing bowls of water in centrally heated rooms.

Indulge in an occasional distilled water rinse. Distilled water is prepared by boiling good, natural water in a closed container, cooling and condensing the resulting steam. Boiled water which has become cold is not distilled water.

IT'S ELEMENTARY

Hair's number one enemies are heat and sunshine. The sun's harsh ultraviolet light waves break down the hair protein, or keratin cells, making the cuticle wither and unable to reflect the light. Hair will become brittle and break. Sunshine fades hair just as it does a pair of shoes in a shop window. Light hair yellows, dark hair fades and bleached or tinted hair can turn to straw. Black hair is an effective block to the sun's rays. The structure of each curl ensures that rays are picked up at several angles and absorbed into the hair, protecting the head and keeping it cool. Yachtsmen take heed, sunshine on its own is perilous enough, combined with wind it's disaster. It lifts the protective cuticle cells leaving the hair looking dull and making it tangly and unmanageable. In sun and wind always wear protective head gear, whether it's a baseball cap or a beret. If not a hat then a good coating of gel or conditioner, washed out in your evening shower, will suffice.

WATER TIGHT

Water acts as a catalyst by speeding up the damaging effects of sun and wind. Salt water and chlorine have drying effects on the hair without help from the elements. Wet hair tangles easily and vigorous combing will result in breakage. Use your protective gel like suntan lotion and re-apply after every dip. Don't tug at hair with a brush when it's wet. Use a wide-toothed comb and if your hair is long, comb a section at a time from the ends and work up to the roots. Tap water contains minerals and salts which determine its degree of hardness. These substances react with soap to form scum which can make hair appear dull and lifeless. Rain and distilled water contain none of these substances and because of their purity are kinder to the hair.

CONSIDERATE CLEANING

"Daily washing of hair should be the rule rather than the exception", states Glenn Lyons, a leading London trichologist. Don't fret about over-washing your hair. It needs to be clean to look good and thrive. This means washing as often as your lifestyle and hair type dictate.

"Compare how you feel", says Elliott Grant, a London barber, "with your best suit on and dirty hair and with jeans and a shirt on but clean hair. Nine times out of ten you'll be more self assured with a clean head of hair no matter how you've dressed your body". The art of clean hair is in the rinsing. An improperly rinsed scalp can cause what you might believe to be dandruff, but is, in fact, scaling. Rinse under the shower or a hand-held shower attachment and concentrate on areas that are easy to forget – behind the ears and the nape of the neck are often neglected. Rinse until you hear the hair squeak with cleanliness. Clean hair will feel polished and smooth when wet and will actually tell you so by making a squeaking noise as you rinse.

DEADLY DRYING

Don't vigorously towel-dry. Towel drying creates heat and heat causes breakage. Blot excess moisture with the towel and if possible allow to dry naturally. Hair appliances and the heat they exude can be deadly adversaries. If the use of a hair dryer is really necessary, first allow the hair to become almost dry naturally. Don't turn the heat up higher than your skin can stand. Although your hair doesn't react to intense heat in the same way your flesh does, it burns just the same. Hold the dryer 10–12 inches away and never concentrate on one area for too long.

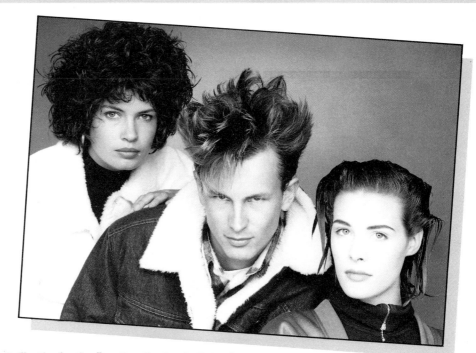

UNNATURAL CAUSES

Chemicals used in perming and tinting can without doubt enhance your hair but handle with care. Wrongly or continuously applied they can change its colour (not for the better), weaken it and, at worst, break it beyond recognition. If you must perm or colour your hair always have it done by an expert. Products designed for use at home are almost identical to those in the salon, but unprofessional application does the damage. If you insist on having such delicate operations performed at home at least engage the talents of a hairdresser to do them. Give your hair a break, don't subject it to a continuous barrage of chemicals. One perm after another will make hair weaker and weaker until eventually it becomes so fine it is unable to hold a perm at all. Allow at least a few months between perms and never have your hair coloured or permed before a holiday in the sun. Sunshine, sand and sea will combine forces with those chemicals to make sure hair sizzles.

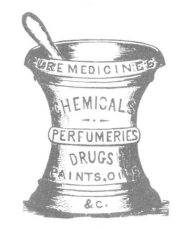

15

FOOD FOR THOUGHT

Your hair is a mirror of your whole well-being. Any adverse conditions – stress, dieting, illness, certain medications – will reflect in your hair. First it will look dull, limp and listless, sometimes scaling (flaking skin) will appear, and hair may even fall out. If the situation is beyond your control – a long illness or course of unavoidable drugs – be patient. Your hair will, with time, recover. But if you can take action you owe it to your hair to do so. Junk food freaks be warned: continue to feed on cheeseburgers and chips and your hair will never shine on. The cells which are busy working beneath your scalp to produce hair need a well-balanced diet to function properly. Omit basic raw materials and production will grind to a halt. Avoid faddy diets: the body will think it's being starved and will save essential nutrients for all the major organs, neglecting hair. Fresh fruit and vegetables are musts. Fish and poultry will help the body thrive. Plenty of water and some fibre will keep the system clean. Cheese is disastrous. It is about the most difficult food for the body to digest and because the metabolism cannot do its work normally, the body doesn't function properly and scaling can result. If real dandruff is your problem, avoid champagne and vintage white wines. Their high sugar content will have an inflammatory effect.

Stress is the greatest cause of temporary hair loss and dandruff. "Stress has a massive influence on the biochemistry of the body", explains a top trichologist, "and this influence is reflected in our external appearance". In some cases stress is unavoidable. But if you can't stop it, ease it. Play sports on a regular basis. Lock yourself in the car and read a book for 30 minutes each day. Take some time for yourself. Relax a little.

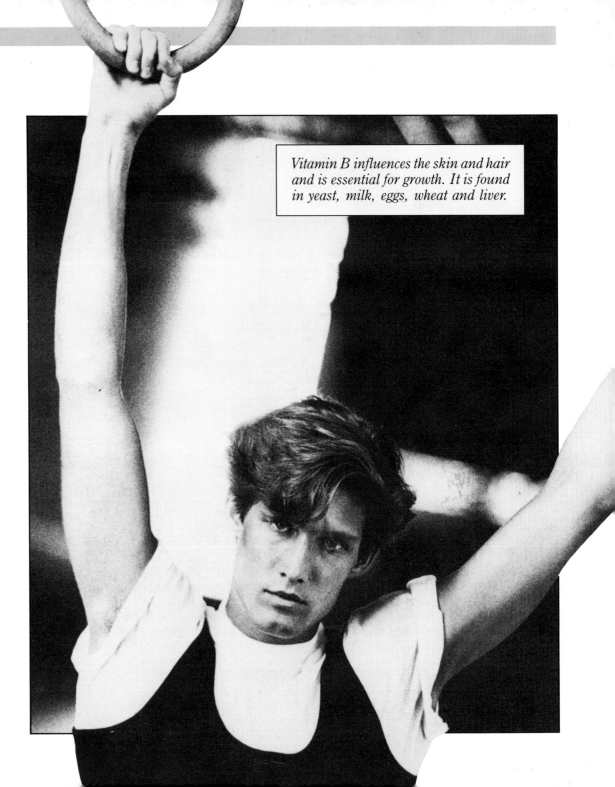

Vitamin B influences the skin and hair and is essential for growth. It is found in yeast, milk, eggs, wheat and liver.

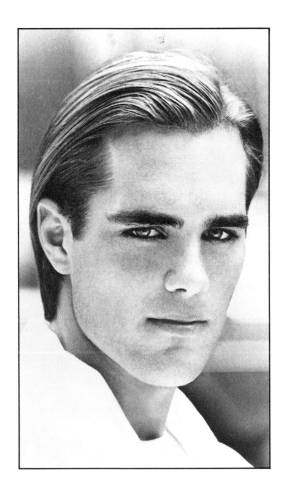

WHAT TYPE ARE YOU?

Get to grips with your hair type. Establish whether it's dry, greasy or a combination of both and why. Root out the cause and find a complementary product, otherwise you could be pouring gallons of expensive, heavy duty conditioner on already over-nourished, greasy hair or starving, dry, brittle hair of the nutrients it so badly needs.

WELL OILED

Excess sebum causes hair to become too greasy too quickly. This happens when the sebaceous glands become over active and swollen, sometimes increasing to three times their normal size. The male hormone testosterone plays a large part in working sebaceous glands overtime and because of this men generally have a tendency towards greasy hair. Greasy hair feels heavy and lank and looks lifeless and dull.

Don't be afraid to wash greasy hair. It's an old wives' tale that frequent washing stimulates the sebaceous glands and makes hair greasy. Hair should be washed as often as it needs to be kept clean and that means at least twice a week, if not every day. When shampooing use lukewarm water, never rub or massage the scalp and do not over-lather. Avoid animal fats, oils and starch and eat plenty of fresh fruit, vegetables and lean meat.

DRY HAIR

This type is brittle in texture and has a dull, almost straw-like appearance. It tangles easily and is unmanageable. Dry hair and scalp are the result of under active sebaceous glands which do not produce enough sebum to lubricate either the scalp or the hair. It is possible to have a greasy scalp and dry hair. This usually happens when the hair has been frequently dried by too hot a hairdryer or been subjected to the sun or chemical processes. Curly hair, and in particular black, afro hair, has a tendency towards dryness. The structure of the curl allows moisture to escape from the hair shaft but it is difficult for sebum to travel down and lubricate hair. Black hair is more brittle as the curls tend to tangle together and the tight bends of the curls cause the hair to open out, fray and break off more quickly than other types.

Protect dry hair at all times from sunshine, get a good "wash and wear" cut that needs little styling. Keep brushing and combing to a minimum. Dry hair needs to be kept just as clean as greasy hair. Every day is probably unnecessary but twice a week is essential. Before you invest in a shampoo check out how your scalp feels. If it is dry you'll need to replace the valuable nutrients of which it is being starved. If your scalp is greasy but your hair dry, approach with caution, look for a combination shampoo and gently cleanse the scalp. If your salon is good, it should be able to sell you a product specifically for this hair type.

MASSAGE MAGIC

If your hair and scalp are really parched, regular scalp massages will help stimulate lazy sebaceous glands. It is a service that might be provided at your salon, or by a trichologist. If you attempt to do it yourself the muscles in your arms will tense and negate the beneficial, relaxing effect the massage should have. Always seek professional advice first. For the massage to be beneficial it is important that the operator knows something about scalp muscles, the system of blood vessels and the network of nerves.

Massage will not only ease tension but stimulate the nerves, muscles and glands in the scalp and increase the circulation of blood which nourishes the scalp tissues. Mixtures of liquid vegetable and mineral oils are usually favoured for body and scalp massage. The operator will divide your hair into sections and work her way from the nape of the neck towards the forehead. By using only the balls of her fingers she will gently but deftly exert pressure and knead the scalp. A good scalp massage should take at least 30 to 40 minutes.

BACK TO NORMALITY

A normal scalp and hair has sebaceous glands which produce just enough sebum for the needs of the hair – not too little, not too much. A normal scalp is common but normal hair, which is ideal and problem free, rare.

WASHING WITH CARE

Whatever your hair type you need to wash your hair regularly. This could mean twice a week or every day. Watch your hair and forget about the myths. If it feels dirty, wash it. Shampooing the hair frees it from everyday pollution like stale perspiration and accumulated dust. But the art of thoroughly cleaning the hair is not as easy as it seems. Insufficient rinsing and the use of too much shampoo are common mistakes but ones which will make your hair feel as if it needs washing again within a very short space of time. There is no short cut to clean hair, but the following guidelines should help:

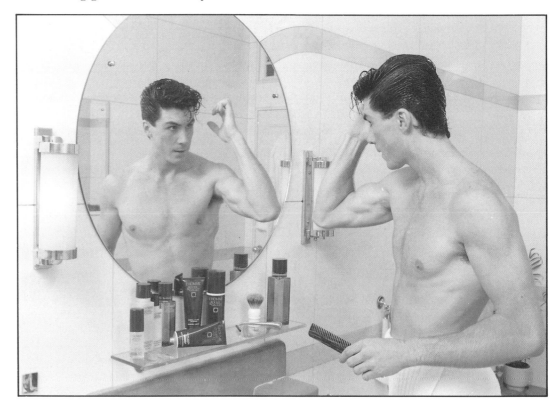

The clean sweep

OR HOW TO GIVE YOURSELF THE BEST SHAMPOO IN THE BUSINESS

1 Brush or comb hair through to loosen dirt and grime and any styling aids which may have been used.

2 Never wash your hair in the bath. How can your hair be clean if it's been rinsed in water tap-high with scum, dirt and grime from your body?

3 Set the shower or tap water lukewarm. A greasy condition will be stimulated by water that's too hot.

4 With your head bent forward, thoroughly soak all the hair.

5 Pour a small amount of shampoo into the palm of your hand and spread it over both palms before application.

6 Gently massage the shampoo into the scalp. Do not be tempted to over-lather or apply more shampoo. The key to a good product is not in the amount of bubbles it makes.

7 Rinse thoroughly. If you shampoo your hair twice a week, repeat the entire process. If you wash your hair every day, one shampoo is enough.

8 Now rinse and rinse again. Concentrate on the areas you might be tempted to forget, like the nape of the neck and behind the ears. Shampoo may loosen the dirt, but it is the rinsing that actually cleans the hair.

9 Blot hair dry with a towel. Hair is at its most fragile when wet so handle with care.

10 Comb style into place with a wide-toothed, saw cut comb and, if possible, allow to dry naturally.

CONDITION WITH CARE

Good marketing has led us to believe that after-shampoo conditioning is essential to any hair care regime. Not so. If your hair is greasy and easy to manage when washed you can probably get away with a slick of conditioner or creme rinse once a week. Dry, brittle hair will lap up much more. After-wash conditioners coat the keratin layers of the cuticle so that they overlap each other, close and lie flat. Hair has less static, becomes smooth and sleek looking and more manageable.

Apply conditioner after you've shampooed and blotted hair dry. Pour a small amount of the product onto the palm of your hand. Spread it over the other palm. Distribute evenly throughout the hair. Do not massage into the scalp, conditioner is for your hair, not your skin. Conditioners usually need to be left on for a couple of minutes to ensure that the cuticles get well coated, use this time to clean any brushes or combs. If the product needs combing through handle with care, remember that hair is at its most fragile when wet. Use a wide-toothed comb and with teeth that lie flat and work it gently through the hair. Rinse thoroughly and wrap a warm towel around the head to blot off excess moisture.

Drying long Victorian hair was such a problem that brushes with hollow teeth, filled with hot water, were invented.

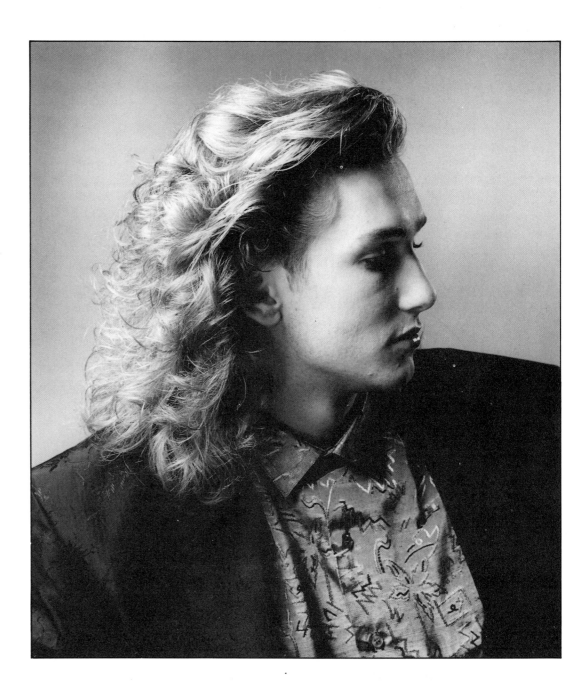

DRY AND DRY

Whenever possible leave your hair to dry naturally. One great advantage you have over women is that shorter haircuts are designed to fall into place naturally where the more contrived styles that women favour tend to need some kind of styling along the way. That inevitably means entering the danger zone of potentially damaging drying tools like hairdryers, heated rollers and hot tongs.

If a hand-held dryer is a must for immaculate styling, look for an appliance with less than 1,200 watts of power. It will eliminate the temptation to dry your hair on too high a temperature setting. Select a dryer with temperature and speed controls and a styling nozzle, so you can control where the heat is going.

Never try and style your hair while it is dripping wet. Hair won't be tackled in such a way while it is soaked, the whole operation will take you twice as long and the style will fall out almost as soon as you've dried it. Give the hair some lift and volume without the use of a hairdryer by finger drying. Simply run your fingers through your hair as if they were a brush. The air distribution created as you move your fingers will enable you to push hair into place.

If you are using a dryer make sure that it is held at least 10 inches away from the head. Keep it constantly on the move to avoid scorching any one patch of hair. Turn off the appliance when hair is throughly dry but allow the hair to cool for a minute or two before you brush or comb through.

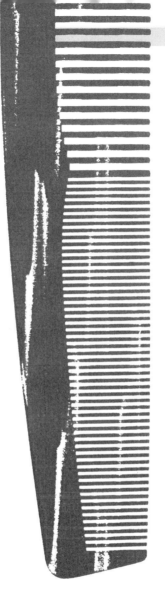

WELL EQUIPPED

The essential tool in any male haircare kit is a comb. Your comb should be capable of arranging your hair and imparting a little fullness without tearing or pulling. Saw cut combs lie flat and smooth and so won't scratch at the hair and cause it to split. Choose a wide-toothed comb to arrange your hair in place while it is wet, it won't snag or tug while your hair is at its most fragile. A finer-toothed comb is more suitable for grooming throughout the day. Remember to clean your comb every time you shampoo. Pollution will be attracted to a dirty comb like bees to a honey pot, particularly if that comb is coated with oil from a greasy scalp.

> *To clean combs wash them in washing-up liquid and give them two rinses, one in water and another in antiseptic mouthwash.*

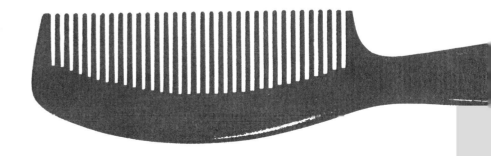

HAIR

BRUSH STROKES

Some experts believe that incorrect brushing can so badly damage the hair they would like to ban the brush altogether. "The use of the wrong brush in the wrong way can cause more damage to the hair than anything else", says a London trichologist, "it can virtually pull hair out by the roots". Most recognize, however, that some brushing is necessary for daily grooming. The answer is to choose your brush wisely and keep the use of it to a minimum. Go for a good name, and whatever size or shape brush you opt for select one with ball-tipped bristles. These will avoid scratching the hair. Some brushes are not only ball-tipped but the bristles are set in a rubber base. This base comes away from the handle easily, making it simple to clean, and because it is made of flexible rubber pulls less at the hair.

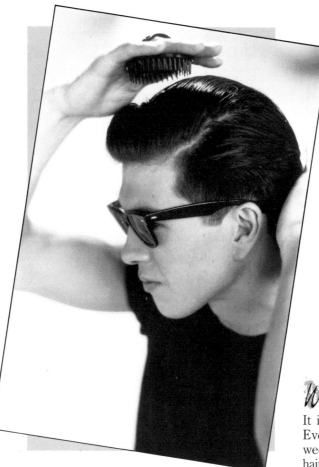

Fingers served as the earliest combs. They were superseded by fish bones fastened between pieces of wood. Greek and Roman women used wood and ivory combs with a double row of teeth for cleaning their heads.

WASH AND BRUSH UP

It is essential to keep hairstyling tools clean. Every time you shampoo is preferable, once a week acceptable. Remove any loose strands of hair from the brush with a wide-toothed comb. Never allow wooden or metal handles to be submerged into the cleansing solution. Immerse the brush, and comb too if you are cleaning them together, in warm soapy water. A few drops of shampoo swished in water will do nicely. Rinse in clean, warm water. Dry the comb and brush handle on a towel and then leave the comb and brush bristles face downwards, on the towel to dry naturally. Don't be tempted to speed things along by putting the brush on a radiator or in strong sunlight – it could become warped.

Common hair problems – at a glance

PROBLEM	DESCRIPTION/CAUSE	SOLUTION
Dandruff	*A skin infection resulting in inflammation of the scalp, some irritation and flaking.*	*A course of special treatment shampoos lasting for several weeks, possibly followed by the application of antiseptic lotions.*
Flaking Scalp	*Often mistaken for dandruff. Caused by infrequent washing and grooming, use of the wrong shampoo, insufficient rinsing, stress.*	*Use a mild shampoo and wash more often. Rinse thoroughly several times, until hair seems to squeak with cleanliness.*
Split Ends	*Harsh brushing, over-use of electrical appliances.*	*Cut them off. Avoid back-combing and use conditioner regularly to help prevent further damage.*
Head Lice	*Contagious parasites which lay their eggs in the hair shaft and live off blood.*	*Your doctor will prescribe a lotion or shampoo for all the household to use. The problem should clear within ten days.*
Dull Hair	*Hair looks dry and lifeless. Possible causes are insufficient rinsing or the adverse effects of chemicals and sunshine.*	*Regular use of after-shampoo conditioner, weekly application of a deep conditioning treatment. Thorough rinsing.*
Frizzy hair	*The result of humidity on curly hair, over-exposure to the elements or over-processing.*	*A shorter, more controllable style. Instant conditioner after every wash.*
Flyaway hair	*Hair's reaction to static electricity in the atmosphere, causing it to stand away from the head out of control.*	*Application of a creme rinse after every shampoo.*
Limp Hair	*Languid hair sometimes caused by inadequate rinsing or by using the wrong product for your hair type.*	*A short cut for bounce and body. Check your products and how you use them, with your stylist.*
Male Pattern Baldness	*Hereditary hair loss. Hair eventually ceases to grow at all. Can result in thinning hair or total hair loss.*	*No cure, just disguises. Consult a trichologist about the alternatives.*

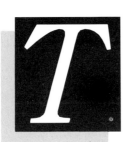

The right stuff

If you are delighted with your haircut but feel let down by its performance between salon visits it could be that you are using the wrong products. Embarrassment, confusion and incomprehension are understandable reactions to the vast number of products available. Look at the bottles, tubs, cans and tubes of hair products for sale on any supermarket, department store or chemist shelf. They all seem so enticing but without any guidance how can you begin to know what is right for you? You may well be tempted to avoid the decision altogether and get the woman in your life to buy your shampoos for you, but does she know exactly what your hair needs?

The best place to ask for advice and narrow the options is your salon. A good salon should retail products because the way your hair looks is a walking advertisement for them, so it is logical that they should be able to sell you products to care for and style it. Most manufacturers produce brands which are sold in salons only. Some believe so strongly that products should only be available in salons and sold through the expert guidance of hairdressers, in the way that doctor's prescriptions are dispensed through pharmacies, that they don't make their goods available to other retail outlets.

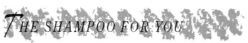

THE SHAMPOO FOR YOU

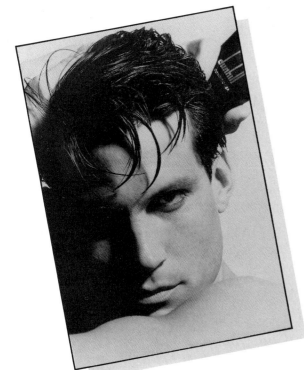

The master of any haircare cupboard is shampoo, which is mainly comprised of detergent, which cleanses the hair. Shampoo also contains thickeners, colourants, preservatives and perfume. Together they work to lift dirt, oil and other foreign bodies off the hair. As a shampoo's performance is most affected by how much detergent it contains, and as this is never listed on the bottle, the only real way of finding out which one works for you is by trial and error. This needn't be as painstaking as it may sound. Buy sachets and trial size bottles until you've found a favourite. Buy a shampoo because it suits your hair type, because you like the way it cleans your hair and because you enjoy using it. Don't buy it for the marketing prose on the back of the bottle. Whatever wonderful added ingredient a shampoo claims to contain, it will only end up being washed down the drain along with the dirt and oil the detergent loosens.

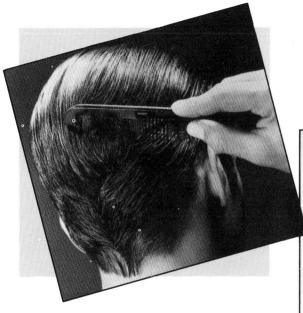

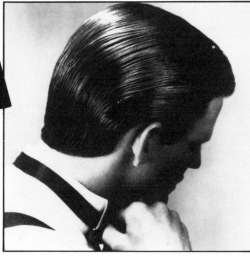

ON CONDITIONERS

Clever marketing has led us to believe that conditioners are absolutely essential after each wash but if your hair is short, easy to manage and has a tendency towards greasiness this isn't true. If, however, your hair is long or dry or needs to be brushed frequently and suffers from static or frizziness, an after-shampoo conditioner, or creme rinse, will help to protect the hair and make it more manageable. Conditioners contain surfactors (detergents) that are attracted to the hair like a magnet by electro-static charges. They work by flattening the keratin scales of the hair shaft and by doing so give it a sleek appearance and make it easy to control.

Protein, or deep-action conditioners, go one step further by actually penetrating through the cuticle into the cortex where they form bonds which help to strengthen the hair and improve its texture. In order to achieve this penetration they are left on the head for longer than creme rinses, usually between 5 and 20 minutes. If your hair is damaged it is prudent to have a conditioning treatment every week. If not, monthly treatments will keep the hair sleek and controllable. It isn't necessary to visit a salon. Protein packs can be purchased in most outlets which retail haircare products and they can be applied in the comfort of your own home.

It is important to remember that no conditioner can perform miracles. Its degree of success in adding gloss and manageability to your hair is purely cosmetic and temporary. It will help damaged hair look healthier than it really is. The only permanent way of restoring life to damaged hair is to cut it off and start again.

THE pH BALANCING ACT

Many shampoos are pH-balanced, which means that like human hair, they are slightly acidic. The pH (or Potential Hydrogen) scale is the rating of a substance's acidity or alkalinity. The scale runs from 0–14 and the middle, number seven, is the point at which acidity and alkalinity balance each other out so that the solution is neutral: distilled water is a good example. Any number below this indicates acidity and above it alkalinity. Hair has a pH level of between 4.5 and 5.5, making it acidic. If your hair has undergone chemical treatments this balance becomes disrupted and harsh alkaline products can weaken the hair shafts and lay them open to

damage. Because of their acidity, pH-balanced shampoos help to make the hair shafts stronger, shinier and more manageable. So if your hair is the least bit damaged it is a pH-balanced shampoo you should be looking out for.

When you are washing your hair don't necessarily follow the instructions on the bottle to the letter. If you are washing your hair more than twice a week, and you should be, you will only need one application of shampoo. If your hair is washed every day look for a frequent use shampoo. These are specially formulated with extra mild detergents which rinse out of the hair easily, therefore decreasing the risk of build-up and a flaking scalp.

FOOD FOR THOUGHT

There is nothing wrong with home-made conditioning treatments and rinses as long as you keep their effect in perspective. Remember that they cannot perform miracles and completely mend the hair. They can also be time-consuming to prepare and messy to use so it might be less frustrating to stick to their ready-made couterparts! Milk, egg whites, beer and other food containing proteins have been used to condition hair. In their natural state they are not very effective conditioners because the size of their protein molecules is too large to penetrate the hair. Like creme rinses however, they can benefit the outside of the hair and help to make it appear healthy. Try this egg conditioning treatment to restore lustre; beat together two eggs and slowly add one tablespoon of olive oil, one tablespoon of glycerine and one teaspoon of cider vinegar. Apply this all over your head once you have shampooed and rinsed your hair and leave the mixture on your scalp for between 15 to 30 minutes. Rinse off well.

HAIR RAISING

Styling aids have been around for a long time but when punks started demanding that their hair levitate for them, and manufacturers met this demand with all manner of sprays, gels and creams to help hair defy gravity, they were thrust from relative obscurity into stardom. Now the selection has become bewildering. Just trying to differentiate between one can of mousse and another can seem like a lifetime's project. Today it's not just punks that wish to preen their hair to perfection. Styling aids play a vital part in creating the versatility that you are demanding of your hair. Before you buy your product, ask your stylist what he or she uses on your hair. If you cannot purchase it in the salon ask what the most similar product is and invest in that. The wrong styling aid can do as much to destroy a new look as the right one can to enhance it.

Brilliantines were once popular dressings which gave an oily surface gloss to the hair. The base was either vegetable or mineral oil. The stiffer variety was thickened with waxes and the liquid variety thinned with spirit. Yardley first manufactured their Lavender Brilliantine in 1920.

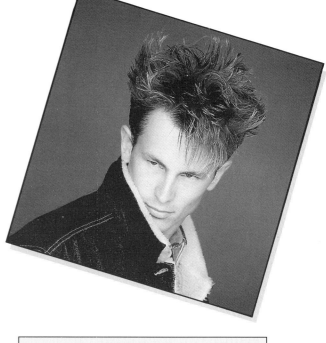

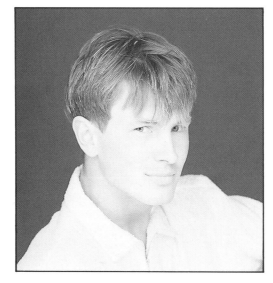

Mousses and gels are chemically very similar. It's the way they are applied which separates them. They are solutions of polymers and resins that set the hair. If gel was thinned and packaged in an aerosol can with propellant it would be a mousse.

For many years Bay Rum was believed to help stimulate hair growth. It became fashionable in the United States in the 19th century and came from crude alcohol obtained during the manufacture of West Indian rum which was then distilled with fresh leaves and berries.

It is the polymers in mousses and gels that effect their staying power. Concentrated, flexible polymers give a stronger hold whilst brittle ones break and brush out easily, resulting in a more gentle hold.

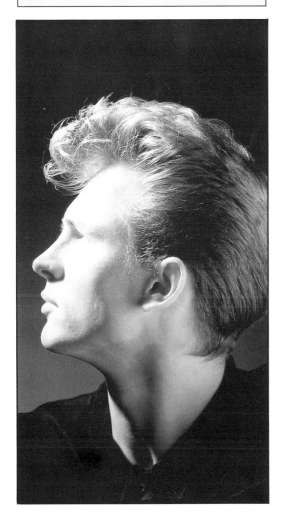

TURN TO A QUIVERING GEL-LY

Gels are clear, concentrated formulas which hold the hair and impart a sheen. They can be used to make hair stand up and give it more bounce or to sleek it down and give it a wet look. A good cut and a tube of gel can be invaluable companions. "Gel is definitely the most versatile styling aid around for men", confirms Elliott Grant of Vidal Sasson's Barber's shop. A mere slick of gel can disguise the side-parted, more conventional style you might wear for the office and transform it into something swanky enough to hold proud down the King's Road. Use a little, rather than a lot of gel at a time to make full use of its build-up potential. Rub a blob between warm palms and work through dry or damp hair. If your hair is fine apply gel only to the roots to avoid hair being weighed down. Too strong a gel can make your hair seem dull so test it first by putting a small amount on the palm of one hand and then rubbing your palms together. A strong gel will stop your hands from coming apart easily and might need to be used on wetter hair to dilute it.

Don't throw away your Brylcreem. More than 60 years after it was first manufactured this gentlemen's grooming aid has enjoyed a comeback. It has been re-launched along with a complementary gel, mousse, Style and Hold Fixing Spray and Modelling Gel. A true success story for the product that, during the last war, was air-dropped to the armed forces to give comforting home thoughts to our boys overseas.

A LOOSE MOUSSE?

Mousse is a hair thickening agent which adds gentle body and volume to the hair. Mousses are especially good for curly hair, which tends to be dry, as they make it slightly oily. Mousse is designed for use on partially dried hair, or on dry hair in between washes to revamp a style. The amount you need to use depends on the length of your hair. A quantity the size of an egg will suffice for most short styles. The longer the hair becomes, the more mousse is needed to mould and control it. Shake the can well, apply a blob of the foam on the palm of your hand and work it all over your head with your fingertips. Then style as usual. Like gels, mousses do vary in strength. Generally, the stickier the mousse feels on your hands the stronger it will hold.

SPRAY ON STYLE

Hairsprays are thin, quick-drying varnishes which leave a transparent, flexible film of resinous material on the hair and in doing so help to preserve the style. They can be sprayed on to your brush or comb and then worked in the hair or sprayed directly on to the finished hairstyle.

The kindest cut of all

Like clothes, hair is something that can boost confidence, but unlike a shirt or jacket, it is much more difficult to change if it doesn't suit. That's why getting the correct style is so important. The key to obtaining the right style for you lies in finding a salon you feel at ease in and a stylist you can communicate with.

If you are having your hair cut at a salon for the first time and the stylist doesn't talk to you before your hair is shampooed, get up and leave. The stylist might create a work of art but he or she cannot possibly know whether it will suit you and your lifestyle unless they have looked at your appearance when you walk into the salon and talked to you then. Assessing your needs when your hair is dripping wet and clinging to your skull isn't on.

SALON STUDY

Start by finding a salon you like the look of and then make a closer study. Analyse what comes out and see whether the looks that are being created are your style. You might want to rid yourself of a few inhibitions but do you really want anything too avant-garde? If there is a friend's hairstyle you particularly admire don't be afraid to ask him where it was done. Very few top salons advertise, new clients are usually recommended by other happy ones. Look for a salon that retails products. If the salon cares about you and the way you look it should care about your appearance between salon visits, and that means guiding you to good shampoos, conditioners and styling aids. It might make your visit more expensive but it will solve the problem of what to choose next time you are faced with the sea of products on the chemist's shelf. Is the salon busy? A good salon should have an atmosphere of organized chaos, bustling yet friendly and efficient. Look for somewhere that offers a free consultation. A stylist meeting a new client for the first time should be prepared to spend a few minutes talking to him about his work, hobbies, what he wants from his hair and what he wants for

him or her. Be prepared to be asked some personal questions and to answer them frankly.

Some British salons bear the mark of good hairdressers: little triangular symbols with *365 Day Hairdressing* on. This is not to say that salons that don't sport this sign aren't good ones, far from it, but members of this organization care enough about their clients to join a club geared towards improving the service and businesses of hairdressers. One great grumble hairdressers have is that clients don't say what they really want, and so go away dissatisfied, never to return. Members of 365 have overcome this by having written plans, almost like personal prescriptions, which are kept as a permanent record of a client's hair. They also contain a home haircare plan which the client takes away. Because you are given these forms to fill in when you arrive at the salon it doesn't matter if you are too shy to speak up, you just write your problems down. The system also means that if you feel confused by all the tips the stylist gives you on cleaning and styling hair, you have something on paper to refer to at home.

It is important to find somewhere you enjoy visiting. We have, after all, progressed a little from medieval times when barbers would also be minor surgeons and tooth-drawers. A haircut should be a more pleasurable experience than that! If you feel nervous about female clients being around, bear in mind they are probably worried about the way they look in your eyes. But if unisex salons are not to your taste look for a barber's shop, not the traditional village variety but the revamped 1980s equivalent. In London, modern barber's shops are booming. Vidal Sassoon, for instance, have been canny enough to recognize that men are demanding more of a service and a domain they can call their own, and have opened several branches. Other barber's shops have firmly established roots in the male market, and the trend is spreading.

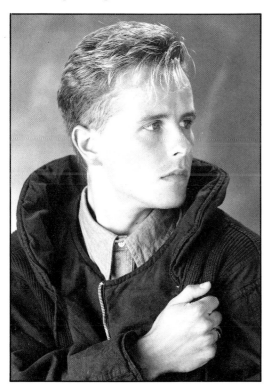

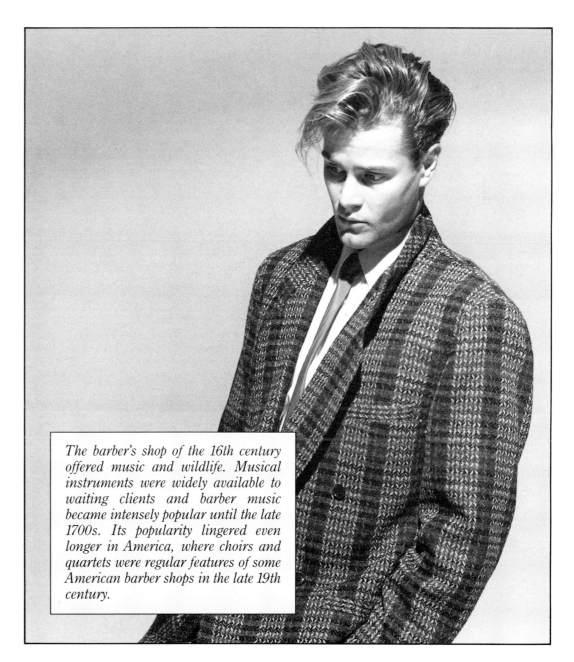

The barber's shop of the 16th century offered music and wildlife. Musical instruments were widely available to waiting clients and barber music became intensely popular until the late 1700s. Its popularity lingered even longer in America, where choirs and quartets were regular features of some American barber shops in the late 19th century.

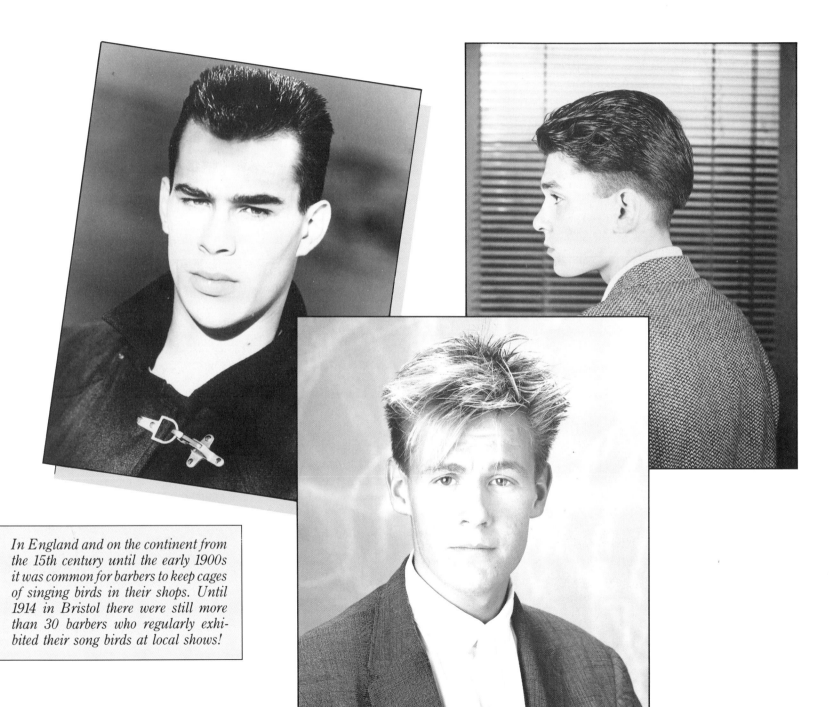

In England and on the continent from
the 15th century until the early 1900s
it was common for barbers to keep cages
of singing birds in their shops. Until
1914 in Bristol there were still more
than 30 barbers who regularly exhi-
bited their song birds at local shows!

USE YOUR STYLIST

Since Vidal Sassoon discovered new hair fashion frontiers in the 1960s the hairdressing industry has undergone a revolution. Hairdressing is no longer a job to fall back on. It's a craft and a career. Today's hairdressers are so highly trained that they have a wealth of knowledge which you should exploit. So talk to them about yourself, allow them to get to know you and realize what you want, draw that knowledge from them. In short, communicate.

"I like to think I encourage my male clients to care more about themselves", says Sharon Dale, a prominent London stylist, "I want them to go away with a fuss-free hairstyle, feeling just a little bit pampered".

A good stylist will not only have undergone three years basic training but will have a career packed full of refresher courses, seminars, shows and late night training sessions. Today's successful stylist cannot get away with a mere flair for hair. He or she needs a lively and friendly personality, a calm temperament, persistence and tenacity to succeed in a job where competition is fierce, fashions are constantly changing and the hours are gruelling. The one thing hairdressers don't have to be is psychic, so if after repeated visits you still haven't said anything about the tuft of hair that annoys you so much you can't blame the stylist. "For the first few salon visits men do tend to be shy", reveals one London hairdresser, "but they don't seem to be as embarrassed by the salon environment as much as they were five years ago. This is because hairdressers are taking the time to teach them about their hair, to show them it really can look great. Look for a hairdresser with a friendly disposition and a good flow of conversation – one who talks to you and thinks of you as a person rather than just another head".

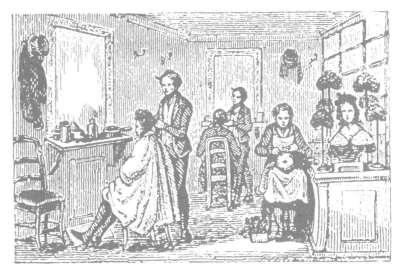

Try and book your appointment for the end of the working day. That way you'll be able to relax without the worry of having to go back to work and the stylist will be able to see you dressed the way you are the majority of the time. Time, it seems, is of the essence with men, and the one thing you won't tolerate is to be kept waiting. "Five minutes", says Elliott Grant of Vidal Sassoon, "is the most you can afford to keep a man waiting. A lady client will sit comfortably for 15 minutes before she becomes agitated". It is understandable that you might be anxious about time if you have to get back to work, but occasionally delays are unavoidable. It only takes a prolonged business meeting to make one male client late and the hairdresser's schedule will be a constant juggle all day. If you do lead a busy working life, book the next appointment as you leave the last one. That way you'll avoid disappointment and annoyance when you phone at the last minute and cannot be fitted in.

"You can't afford to make a mistake with a male client because if you do, you've lost him forever", says Elliott Grant. Hairdressers are in agreement, there are no second chances where men are concerned. One slip up and you never return to the salon again. As Elliott Grant finds, "A displeased male client is the worst there is". There is no room for amateurs in hairdressing these days and you have every right to demand the best. But if you are displeased with the results, why not try talking out the problem with the stylist? See if you can get it right next time. We all have off days and make mistakes. The whole art of getting hairdressing to work for you lies in communication. If you don't tell your stylist what is wrong he or she will never know. But it seems that once you have found someone who really works for you and your hair you remain faithful and sometimes become friends for life. "Women often change their hairdresser on a whim", reveals Sharon Dale of Stephen Way's Bond Street salon, "a man would never do that. Once he's got what he wants he sticks with it. A happy man is putty in your hands, a trusting and devoted client".

BEYOND THE FRINGE

Although face shape and bone structure dictate to a certain extent what your hairstyle should be there are much more important, and less visible factors that should influence the style of your hair: your personality and the life you lead. It's no good, for instance, growing your hair to your shoulders if you work in a bank and play a lot of squash. It might look fantastic, but sporting something so fashionable and high profile might alarm the bank's customers and it won't be too long before it starts annoying you on the squash court.

The stylist can read a lot from the way you look when you enter the salon. If you walk in on a Saturday morning wearing jeans and a denim jacket, looking casual and arty, that's the person the style will be created for. Yet if you spend 80 per cent of your time in an office with a suit on that style is bound to be wrong. That's why it's so important to dress the way you normally do for a salon visit.

A good cut is the essence of healthy, happy, hassle-free fair. "Men don't want the bother of a fussy hairstyle", reports Elliott Grant "very few salons will use a blow-dryer on a man's head these days because they recognize the fact that men can't be bothered with all that". A good cut should be easy to handle and versatile. It should bounce back into place after a wash and maybe a lick of mousse or gel. It shouldn't let you down between salon visits. What's the use of a haircut if it only looks good once every six weeks? If you know you are doing something wrong when styling at home but can't quite put your finger on it, go back to the salon and demand to be shown how to handle the style again.

Photographs are always encouraged in salons to help establish what you want. But be realistic. All the styling aids and cutting techniques in the world aren't going to mould hair into a position nature didn't intend for it. If you have greasy hair avoid anything too face framing. Those oily strands of hair can fall into your face and cause unnecessary blemishes. Don't try and compensate for fine, wispy hair by growing it, it will look stringy rather than stunning. Very dry hair is best kept in good condition with a short, sharp shape. Grow it too long and it can become brittle and cause split ends. Very curly hair becomes heavy as it grows longer and can lose its shape. Have it cut to enhance your facial features, keep it short and maintain its natural bounce.

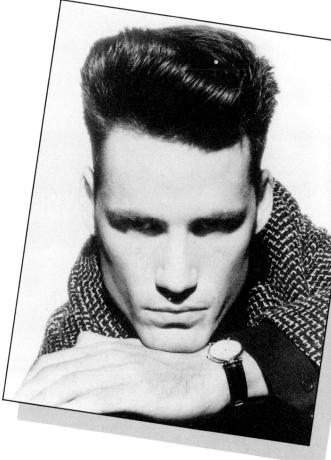

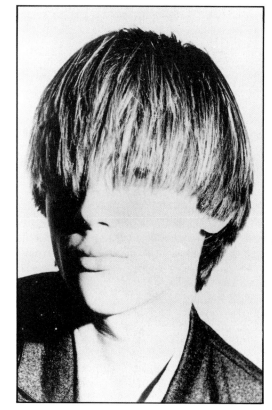

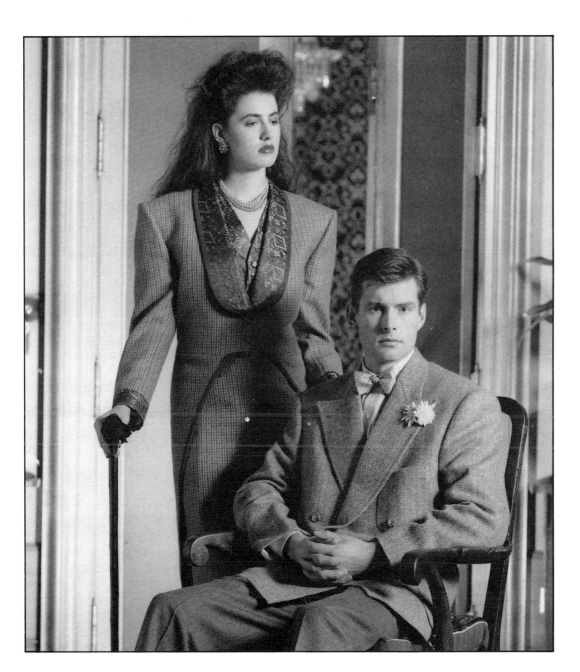

UNDER THE INFLUENCE

Wife, mother, mistress, secretary or daughter, there's a woman out there who has an influence on the way you look. 'A man's appearance is totally dictated by the women in his life", echoes Elliott Grant. It is not uncommon for a wife to go into the salon with her husband to make sure the stylist doesn't cut off a fraction too much!

Take a long, hard look at yourself. She may love your hair the way it's been for years but what does everyone else think? Do you feel that it brings out the best in you and boosts your confidence? If your hairdresser has been urging you to try something a little different seriously consider what he or she says. "Men will tread carefully rather than go in for the kill", one hairdresser admitted. "The wife of one male client threatened to break both my legs if I permed her husband's hair. I value my legs too much to try and win her round".

If you want to bring a breath of fresh confidence into your life think about changing your hairstyle, no matter how subtly. Relax your attitudes a little and don't take high fashion looks too seriously. They are meant to be taken from magazines and watered down to suit the individual. There are alternatives to punk, pink and vertical, as there are to the classic short, back and sides.

*T*hrough thick and thin

No matter how much care you take of your hair it is still possible to have problems. One of the most irritating hair complaints of all is dandruff. The bad news is that there are seventeen known types of dandruff of which two, dry and greasy dandruff, are the most common. The good news is that even if your scalp is shedding little white flecks all over your best navy suit you probably haven't got either of these but are suffering from a flaking, or scaling, scalp.

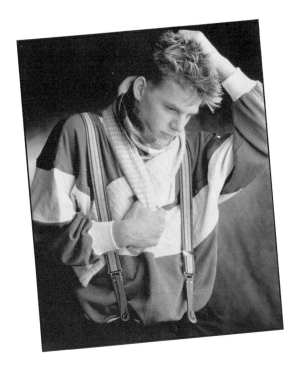

*R*EAL DANDRUFF

Real dandruff is a skin infection caused by the skin's natural antiseptics and defensive mechanisms being overcome by infectious organisms. It is characterized by a mild inflammation of the scalp and the formation of a deposit which consists of grey, or yellowish, scales about the size of a match-head. Irritation may or may not be present.

Dry dandruff can be found on dry, greasy and normal scalps. It is a fungus which infects the top layer of the skin causing it to build up and flake excessively. These flakes then fall through the hair. Greasy dandruff is only found on greasy scalps and is non-scaly. The infectious organism travels quickly down the layers of the skin, feeding off cells which are alive as it does so. The flakes are invisible because they are flattened and held on the scalp by sebum. The solution to real dandruff is usually a five or six week course of special treatment shampoos, possibly followed by the application of antiseptic lotions. These can be "prescribed" by a good hairdresser but you can also consult your doctor or trichologist. These products will work by penetrating the bottom layer of the skin where living cells are constantly being produced. Avoid rubbing the scalp unnecessarily, it will only make the irritation worse, and keep brushes and combs scrupulously clean.

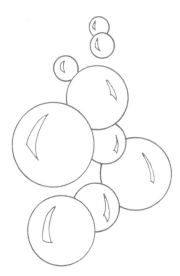

FALSE DANDRUFF

When it comes to a flaking scalp, or false dandruff, you may have to blame yourself as it is often the result of poor hair. Infrequent grooming and washing, too harsh a shampoo used too often and insufficient rinsing can all cause a flaking scalp. Stress can also be the culprit.

In order to cure this malady it is essential that you allow more time for your hair. A dip in the bath or quick rinse under the shower are not the way to a clean, healthy head of hair. A flaking scalp will continue unless hair is rinsed properly. Use a milder shampoo more frequently than you normally do and work clean (not bath) water through your hair with your fingers. Guide it through the worst affected and often neglected areas and rinse four times more than you think you should.

If you've done all this and the problem still hasn't cleared up then its probably stress related. "Stress", admits London trichologist Glenn Lyons, "is one of the biggest causes of false dandruff. Stress has a massive influence on the biochemistry of our bodies and this is bound to upset our external appearance, which is only a mirror of the inner self". Attempt to relieve the tension and stress of everyday life by playing sport or taking up a hobby for a couple of hours a week. Your hair will benefit along with the rest of your body!

SPLITTING HAIRS

Split ends are less of a cause for concern to men than women as the major causes, harsh brushing, and over-use of electrical styling appliances, aren't usually necessary with men's styles. Split ends are also more common with long hair than with short. Longer, older layers of the hair shaft tend to separate and split more easily.

There is no magic solution to the split ends saga. There are no lotions, potions or treatments which will stick the ends back together and make them stay that way. The only way to get rid of them is to have them cut off. If you are prone to split ends don't be tempted to tug away at tangles from the root to the ends of your hair. Start at the bottom and gently work your way up.

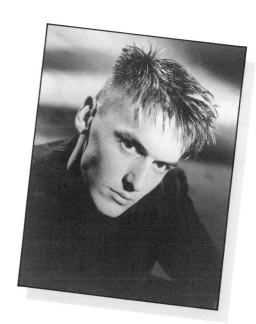

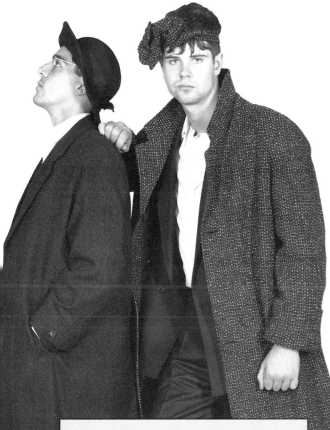

If head lice are left to go too far, they can make a person prone to infection and lethargy. The term nitwit comes from the dozy effect head lice had on their victims in days gone by.

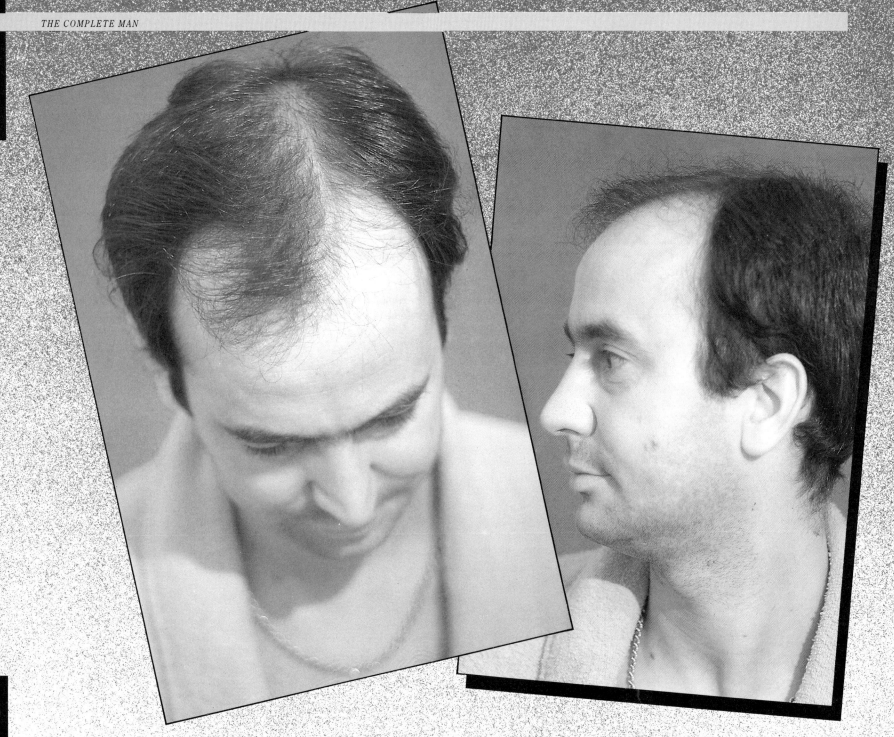

Head Lice

If you are the smartest city gent with clean, short hair, don't think you are immune to head lice. They'll love you. They are no respectors of class, income bracket, sex, age or cleanliness. The chances are that if you have children of school age, your family will fall foul of head lice at some stage. Head lice are parasites which live off blood. A louse is about two millimetres in length, has a triangular head, an oval body and three pairs of legs. The female can lay more than 50 eggs into the hair shaft, at the same time secreting a cement-like substance which adheres to the eggs very near the scalp. After about six days the egg will hatch and the newborn louse will travel into the scalp to reach the blood.

Luckily lice are easy to detect and can be treated at an early stage. Apart from itchiness, particularly at the back of the head, you should be able to see the eggs. These are pear-shaped little masses, firmly attached to individual hairs and close to the scalp. Your doctor will prescribe a lotion or shampoo and the problem should clear up within about ten days. Head lice are contagious, so it is vital that even if only one member of the family has them, the rest of the family should be treated.

Dull Performance

There are less irritating problems than dandruff or head lice which can still adversely affect the hair's performance. Dull hair can result from insufficient rinsing or from the drying effects of chemicals and sunshine. Make an instant conditioner or creme rinse part of your haircare regime. Use it after every shampoo. It will smooth over rough layers of hair, help the cuticles to lie flat, so that the hairs reflect the light and restore sheen. Put on extra gloss with a more penetrating, deep-action conditioner or protein pack once a week. Make sure any conditioner is thoroughly rinsed out and as a final rinse try adding two tablespoons of white vinegar to a quart of water and pouring it over your hair to make sure that every trace of shampoo and conditioner has been removed.

Frizzy and flyaway hair can both be helped with the regular use of an after-shampoo conditioner. Flyaway hair is the result of its reaction to static electricity in the atmosphere and a creme rinse will help to reverse this electrical charge on the hair shaft. Frizzy hair can be the result of humidity on curly hair (go into a sauna with an uncovered, permed head of hair and see the frizzles fly), or hair damaged by over-processing or exposure to the sun and wind. An instant conditioner will help control the frizzles by making the hair easier to manage. If damage is excessive the only certain cure is to have all the damaged hair cut off – that may mean cutting out a new perm which has been over exposed to the elements.

Hair Today and Gone Tomorrow

The most common problem any hair specialist sees in men is hair loss. It may be temporary, like Alopecia Areata, a stress-related complaint where hair falls out in patches, or the more common, and permanent, Male Pattern Baldness. Male Pattern Baldness can manifest itself as just a thinning of the hair or complete lack of hair over the whole or greater part of the scalp. MPB is hereditary and there is absolutely nothing you can do to prevent it. If your father was bald by the time he was 40, don't panic. MPB isn't necessarily passed down from generation to generation nor will it happen to the same extent in each generation.

The male sex hormone androgen causes MPB as it shortens hair's growth cycle. Hair no longer grows for a period of two to six years but for a shorter time, and each successive cycle becomes shorter. If you have MPB you will first notice the hair on top of your head failing to grow to any appreciable length. Finally, only a short fuzz is seen.

It is possible that your hair may appear to be falling out when actually it isn't. Try to remember that hair is constantly going through a growing, resting and shedding cycle. It is bound to appear to fall out more at some periods than at others. This is probably because it has finished its life cycle. After a resting period of about three months a new hair normally forms in the hair follicle, initiating a new growth cycle. If the old hair is still present the new hair will push it out. About 15 per cent of hairs scattered throughout the scalp are in the resting stage and gradually shedding. It is these hairs you may find on your pillow, in the wash basin, and on your brush and comb. Everyone loses hair everyday. Sometimes as many as 100 hairs are shed in a 24 hour period.

Remember that this rate of hair loss is quite normal – it is only when the rate of loss exceeds the rate of growth that thinness and baldness become apparent. This happens as you grow older and some permanent thinning of hair is inevitable with age. But at least 40 per cent of your hair must be lost before thinning is noticeable.

American Indians are reputed to have once eaten sunflower seeds to improve the texture of their hair and add gloss to those long, dark locks.

BALD CAN BE BEAUTIFUL

You can slow down the process of Male Pattern Baldness by treating your hair with care and consideration and by avoiding harsh chemical treatments, but you cannot avoid the end result. There is no cure. Lotions, potions and ointments do not work. If a product is advertised as working wonders it is probably because it has been used on a temporary hair loss situation, like Alopecia Areata.

The best alleviation for MPB is psychological. Try and accept the situation and make the most of it – it can even be enjoyable. "Bald doesn't have to be bad", says Joshua Galvin, prominent hairdressing figure, and he should know, he started losing his hair at the age of 18. "I've simply never worried about it", he adds, "I've always thought that camouflage can be far more ageing than any degree of baldness".

There are ways of looking good, even with very little hair. Confront your hairdresser with your problem, you'll probably find him helpful and sympathetic. The worst thing you can do is grow your hair long on one side and purposely comb it over your head to disguise a bald crown. One whisper of a breeze, all will be revealed and your hair will look unkempt.

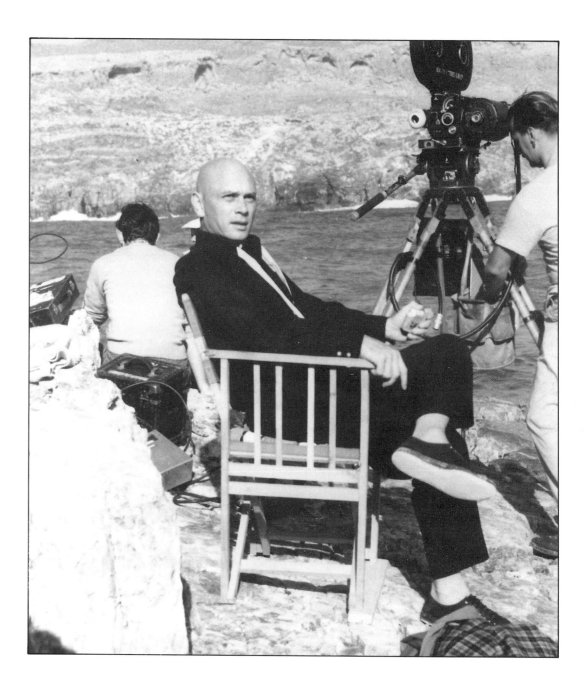

THE LONG AND SHORT OF IT

To make the most of your hair try and achieve some balance. There is little point in growing your hair long at the back if you are totally bald on the crown. The length will only draw more attention to your less plentiful areas, as will long sideburns grown to compensate for hair loss. All they will do is make it more obvious. "I always have a sympathetic ear for my balding clients", reveals one busy stylist, "I try and encourage them to exploit what little they've got rather than camouflage it. If, for instance, a client was going bald on top I'd probably cut the sides and back short so that he looked smart and neat". Wise words. Shorter hair is bouncier because it has no weight to pull it down. It therefore stands up better and looks more abundant. Have a little length left on the collar to add softness to your jawline. Take your height into consideration. If you are of less than average height you cannot afford to have your hair cut too close to the crown as thinning will be more obvious to taller people. Whatever you do don't despair. Hair loss doesn't necessarily mean that your stylist will lose interest in you. Ask for help and try and work it out together.

GOING, GOING, GONE

If you simply cannot learn to accept hair loss, there are ways of overcoming the problem but some of them are pretty gruesome, downright uncomfortable, or both. "I will do my utmost to convince a man that hair loss needn't ruin his life", says leading trichologist Glenn Lyons, "but if it shatters his confidence to such an extent that he cannot lead a normal life I will tell him of the alternatives and advise him on what to do and where to go".

TRANSPLANTS

The most successful, effective and expensive alternative is a hair transplant. This is a surgical operation but it is permanent. Once your new, transplanted hair grows you can do anything with it. For transplantation to be effective hair loss needs to have reached its peak. If you have a transplant at the age of 25 and then lose twice as much hair again in the succeeding five years the transplanted hair is going to look oddly abundant and you'll need another operation to rectify this. So if you are under 30, hang on to what you've got for the time being.

IMPLANTS

An implantation is where anchor points or stitches are inserted into the scalp and hair pieces attached to them. This method carries most risk of infection. It is very difficult to clean adequately under the hair piece, the scalp is constantly under pressure as the hair is groomed and daily grooming loosens the stitches, eventually causing them to fall out and making it necessary to repeat the whole procedure. The scalp won't tolerate that much abuse. "I have seen a man's head so covered in pus after an implantation", warns Glenn Lyons, "that it has become completely yellow and so painful that it was unbearable for him to go out walking on a breezy day".

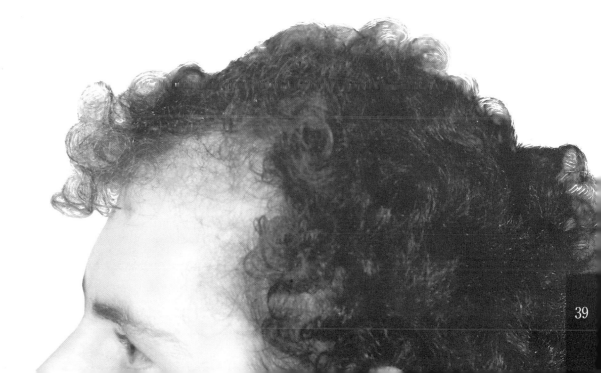

LOOSE WEAVE

A less gruesome way of wearing a hair piece, but one which puts the existing hair under a great deal of stress, is the weaving method. For·this you must have some natural hair growth which is woven or knotted to form anchor points. False hair is either sewn, woven or glued into these anchor areas and then trimmed or styled to blend with the natural hair. The main problem with this process is that as the natural anchor hair grows the hair piece becomes loose, making it necessary to have the hair piece tightened every six weeks or so. This puts the natural hair under tremendous pressure and can result in the temporary baldness known as Traction Alopecia, loss caused by the hair being pulled tight over a long period of time.

Other points to watch: Colour match can be difficult, and a bad match can look like a rug on top of the head. Keeping the scalp under the piece clean isn't easy as it is difficult to get at, yet if it isn't done properly, infection can result.

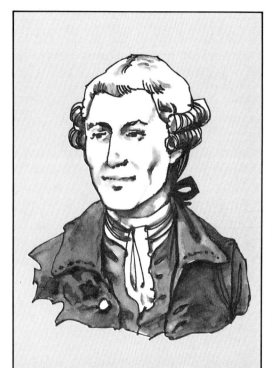

The powdering of wigs became fashionable around 1715 when it was realized that the preferred, pre-bleached, lighter wigs soon became discoloured. People began to use powder made from finely ground starch or wheat flour scented with orange flower, lavender or orris root. In 1795 the government needed to finance the wars against France and so introduced a tax on powder. Those who powdered had to have a certificate for which the fee was one guinea per year – although concessions were made for fathers with more than two unmarried daughters!

TOUPÉE OR NOT TOUPÉE

Wigs and hairpieces are certainly less complicated alternatives to transplants, implants and weaves but it is crucial to get the fitting and colour right if you want to avoid them looking like spare parts. Nothing looks worse than a wig which is a totally different colour from that of the natural hair. Remember that your hair loses pigment with age and your skin becomes more sallow. Choose a wig or piece one or two shades lighter than when your hair was at its most prolific. Before you lash out on the expense of a wig, bear in mind that wearing something so totally alien to your head for such long periods of time takes a lot of getting used to. It can be hot, itchy and uncomfortable, a bit like wearing a hat all day.

Don't turn to any of these alternatives though, without first seeking the advice of a trichologist. Your hairdresser should be able to refer you to one but if not, look up your nearest practice or trichological clinic in your local directory. A qualified trichologist not only possesses in-depth knowledge of hair, skin and scalp but is trained in the preparation of hair products and is able to treat hair and scalp maladies. He has to pass examinations in chemistry, physics, anatomy, microscopy and physiology. If he is unable to convince you that bald can be beautiful he can at least advise you where to go for help, recommending only the best surgeons and expert wig makers. Many ill-fitting wigs and bad weaves are the result of cowboy outfits which set up shop to make a fast buck, caring not a jot about whether your hair piece suits you, your scalp is healthy or your confidence boosted.

In 1624 Louis XIII of France went prematurely bald. He disguised this with a wig and started a fashion that lasted for over 150 years.

A short hair style was adopted by the Duke of Bedford in 1795 to counter the tax on hair powder. It was sometimes called the "Bedford Level".

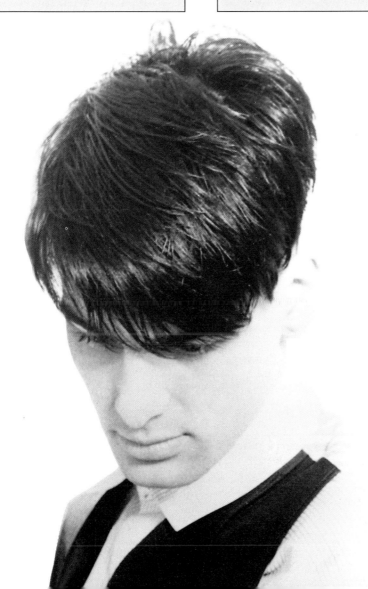

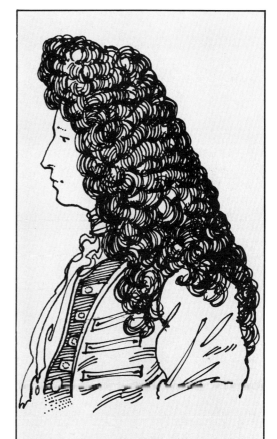

Sir Cloudesley Shovell, a late 17th century Admiral, wore a full-bottomed wig with a mass of tight curls framing his face. The wig named after him was large and flamboyant with cascades of curls falling to below the shoulders. Since only the rich could afford the luxury and expense of buying and maintaining these wigs, the name "big wig" came to be applied to men of wealth and importance.

Wave upon wave

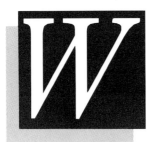

THE PERMANENT SOLUTION

If you've never considered a perm the chances are you've dismissed the idea as effeminate. But the perming process has been revolutionized and refined to such an extent that the whole chemical reaction is not only much kinder to the hair than it was at the turn of the century, when professional perming methods were first introduced, but also much more discreet. "At least 40 per cent of the perms we perform on men are undetectable" says Elliott Grant, top vidal Sassoon barber, "the days of the footballer's, curly-all-over perm have well and truly gone." Hairdressers now focus on designing hair styles for the individual rather than following set trends and because of this partial perming techniques are employed, giving a style lift and body where the hair needs it most rather than perm the whole head of hair. Perms can now go virtually undetected and be an absolute boon if you have a section of hair that seems particularly limp and reluctant to perform the way you'd like it to. A perm can enhance a style, make the hair appear more profuse and, if your hair is greasy, can dry it out a little.

GROWTH PATTERN

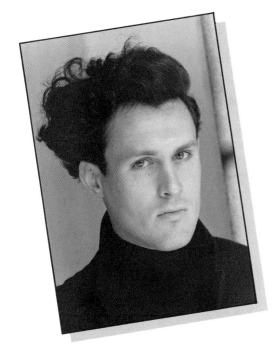

Permanent waves are just that: permanent. But as the hair grows the perm grows down with it and eventually gets cut off. A perm can last for almost a year if you never have your hair cut during that time, but if you have regular trims every four to six weeks the perm will gradually be cut out after three or four months. Women tend to hang on to their locks for a greater length of time than men, generally pre-ferring longer, softer styles. Men's shorter styles can be an advantage because frequent cutting means there is far less risk of old, permed hair becoming dry, split and unmanage-able.

The Machine Permanent method of waving hair introduced in 1905 required electricity to heat large metal clamps that were placed over the client's hair.

Perming is a chemical process which re-forms the structure of the hair and the end result is entirely dependent on the size of the perm roller used, not on the strength of the perming lotion. Leaving the perm lotion on for too long will make no difference to the perm's staying power.

PERMANENT PRECAUTIONS

It is important to remember that perming is a delicate operation that needs to be skilfully performed. Never consider using a home perm kit. If you are embarrassed about having such a process done in a salon or want to cut costs then forget about a perm, your hair should be more valuable to you than that. It is not the perm lotion that produces bad results (such as brittleness, frizziness, split ends and breakage), but the way in which it is applied. Keeping the hair at a constant temperature is an important part of the perming process and at home it is easy to sit in a draught or to walk from the heat of one room to another, perhaps to answer the telephone. By doing this you could end up with one part of your perm "taking" more than the other, with disastrous results.

If you are considering a perm be honest with your hairdresser about the products you've been using on your hair. Any kind of colourant, even those your best friend could not detect, could spell disaster if a perm is applied on top of it. There are perms which can be used on chemically treated hair, but as a general rule if your hair is coloured it is best to steer clear of any more chemical treatments as the risk of damage will become greater.

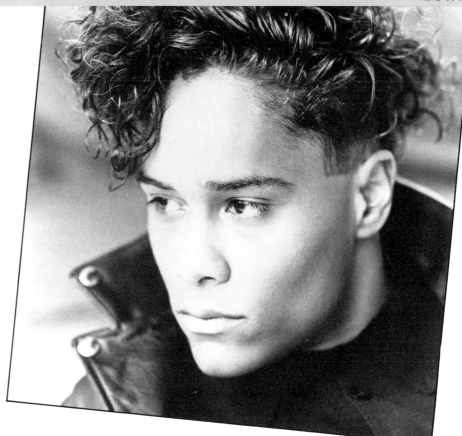

WHAT IS A PERM?

There are many professional perms to choose from. Your stylist will find the right one for your hair. Some look different during application, some feel more comfortable and others claim to be kinder to the hair. The popular Exothermic perm, for instance, has a relatively low pH and is therefore kinder to the hair, making it ideally suited to hair which might already be slightly damaged. But it was the cold wave which revolutionized the industry in 1940 and still remains the firm favourite today. The cold wave was the first method of use chemicals, rather than heat, to perm hair.

The Cold Wave works with the use of waving solution, neutralizer, rods (or perm curlers) and end wraps. The perm lotion works by breaking the hair's sulphur bonds, which maintain its shape. Lotion is usually applied after hair has been wound around rods. Wraps or papers are placed on the end of each hair strand to protect and control it as it is being wound. The broken bonds will now reform around the rod taking on its shape, or diameter. After 10 or 20 minutes the newly formed curls must be locked into shape by the neutralizer. The neutralizer hardens and shrinks the hair shaft and stops the action of the waving lotion. Assuming that you are having your hair cut and styled with your perm, the whole process should take around two hours.

HAIR

PERMING PITFALLS

Adverse reactions to permanent waving are pretty rare these days and when they do occur they are usually the result of lotion or neutralizer inexpertly applied or hair that is subjected to one perm after another. The most common complaints are brittleness, frizziness, split ends and breakage close to the scalp. These can be the result of the waving solution being left on too long or the hair being neutralized inadequately. If your hair is fine or limp it will be pretty resistant to permanent waving and will need a fairly strong lotion to counteract this. Dry, brittle, damaged hair will also be resistant as well as prone to further damage, so special care will be required. To avoid having a perm which lets you down and damages your hair always consult a hairdresser about whether or not you should have a perm and if so, what sort. If your hair is in good condition to start with, the chances of it suffering after a perm are remote. So invest in regular weekly intensive conditioning treatments at least two weeks before your perm and never, ever, have your hair permed and coloured on the same day. If you insist on undergoing both processes, allow at least a week between them.

Allergic reactions can result from a perm, especially if the lotion is allowed to trickle onto your skin during processing. To avoid this make sure that your hairline is thoroughly padded by absorbent cotton wool and that there is a towel around your neck to catch any drips. If either your towel or cotton wool become wet, say so and insist that they are replaced and if any lotion runs onto your face or neck during processing despite these shields, dab it off immediately.

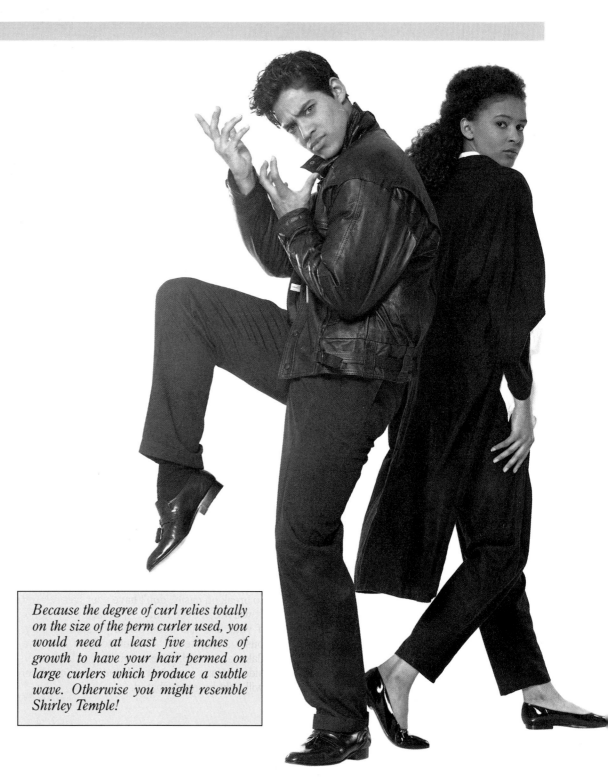

Because the degree of curl relies totally on the size of the perm curler used, you would need at least five inches of growth to have your hair permed on large curlers which produce a subtle wave. Otherwise you might resemble Shirley Temple!

CARING FOR YOUR PERM

Don't leave the salon until you've consulted your hairdresser about what products you should be using on your hair. The hair's structure has been changed, broken down and rebuilt again, and the shampoo you used before your perm might not be the correct one to use afterwards.

Invest in a conditioner. Use a creme rinse after every wash and a deep acting conditioning treatment once a week if possible. These will help you make the most of that perm by retaining lustre and manageability.

Always use a hat or protective barrier cream or gel to guard against the drying effects of the elements and keep the use of electrical appliances down to an absolute minimum.

Have your hair cut regularly to keep its bounce. Add extra bounce and bolster the remaining perm with the help of a styling gel or mousse.

Ask your stylist's advice on how to use these styling aids to your advantage.

Hair should not be permed more than once every four months.

STRAIGHTEN UP

Straightening is essentially the whole perming process in reverse. Many people with a naturally abundant head of curls long for straight hair which is generally easier to manage and more versatile. Black, afro hair forms such tight curls that it can start to grow into the skin, irritating the follicles and making the scalp inflamed. Straighteners help this problem by turning the curls away from the scalp and preventing these ingrown hairs.

Chemical straightening and chemical relaxing are two different processes which produce different effects on the hair. Chemical straightening is the relaxing of naturally wavy hair and chemical relaxing is the relaxing of tighter, kinky, curly hair. Straightening can relax naturally wavy hair without breaking it but it is not strong enough to relax really curly hair in a short time. Whatever the process, take heed, straightening is potentially the most dangerous process that can be performed on a head of hair and it is very difficult to make very curly hair totally wave-free without excessive risk. When hair is permed, the waving lotion is applied after it has been wrapped in curlers. The application is therefore controllable and little of the chemical is likely to come into contact with the scalp. When hair is straightened the lotion is applied all over the scalp, increasing the chances of skin irritation.

If your hair is dry, brittle, damaged or tends to break off easily, don't have your hair relaxed. It will break even more. Approach with caution if your hair has been colour treated or previously straightened. If your scalp is sensitive, flaky, scratched, sore or tender don't even consider having your hair relaxed. Your condition will only be exacerbated.

Pomades were the earliest methods of controlling extremely curly hair. The original ingredients were pig's lard and apples but various animal and vegetable bases were used later, scented with flower oils. They worked by plastering the hair against the scalp and, because they were more effective on short hair, were generally used by men rather than women.

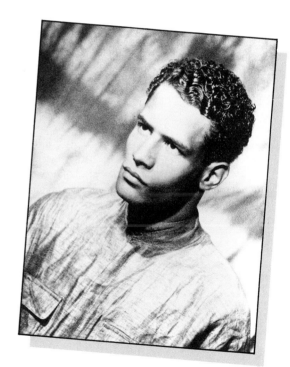

Dyeing for it

If the thought of having your hair coloured makes you turn red with embarrassment, don't worry, colouring techniques have become so refined, simplified and diverse that there is no need to spend hour after tedious hour in the salon or to be shackled to the colourist's brush to have your roots "touched up" every couple of weeks. The industry realized a long time ago that if women hated such a chore, men simply wouldn't tolerate it, and techniques have been refined to such an extent that there seems to be no end to the ways in which you can add a touch of colour and class to your hair. Colouring is by far the easiest and most effective way of polishing a good cut to perfection and there are so many methods available that it needn't be the commitment it once was. Hair colour, no matter how subtle, can bring out the best in a good cut and is an ideal way of covering grey hair.

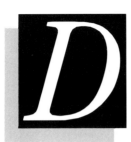

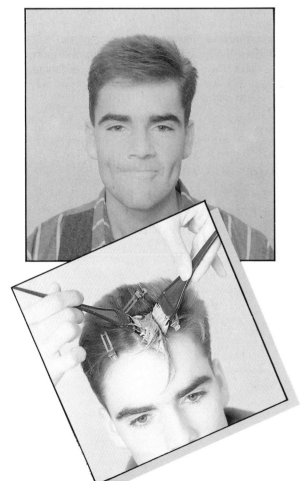

There is no scientific evidence to support tales of hair going grey overnight. Normal greying is part of ageing and is slow but progressive. Hair turns grey gradually, when the pigment cells become inactive. The cells work near the root to deposit pigment in the hair shaft as it forms. When hair turns grey or white it is because these pigment cells have become dormant. So although future hair will not be coloured, those hairs already visible are not affected.

Colourants basically fall into three categories: temporary, semi-permanent and permanent. Colour is the final stage in the creation of a new hairstyle and is applied after a perm if a perm is necessary. In the case of men's shorter hair, colour can give all the lift and texture a style needs, eliminating the need for a perm altogether.

Temporary colour

Temporary colours are the wash-out variety. They only stay in the hair until the next shampoo. They penetrate no further than the hair cuticle, which they thinly coat. They come and go in many shapes and forms, some of which have purely novelty value. The most popular are rinses, which contain combinations of chemicals and colours made from vegetables and herbs. If you are young and unconventional coloured mousses and gels are a fun way of experimenting with temporary hair colour. They are

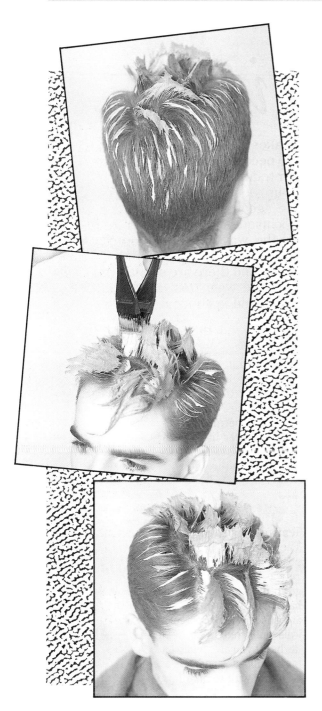

available in an array of dazzling colours, as well as the more subdued ones, can be combed through the hair for a highlighted effect or literally sprayed on for a more outrageous, party look – and they wash out in your next shampoo. Spray-on glitter colours are particularly effective for night life.

SEMI-PERMANENTS

These partially penetrate the cortex and actually put some colour inside the hair. Semi-permanents contain chemicals which raise the pH level to an alkaline range of between seven and nine which causes the cuticle to swell, giving the colour an opportunity to enter the cortex. Once there, the sulphur molecules which contain the colour pigment hang on to the hard protein fibre (keratin) of the cuticle and some of the salt bonds in the cortex, staining the cuticle and partially colouring the cortex. As penetration of the cortex is not complete, the colour will fade rather than grow out. This usually takes between four and eight shampoos.

Although this type of colour washes out fairly quickly, particularly if you shampoo daily, you can create a build-up effect. Re-apply the colour at frequent intervals – weekly or fortnightly depending on your normal hair care routine – and the colour will become richer rather than fade. Semi-permanents cannot lighten the hair as they contain no bleaching agents but they are ideal for enriching natural hair colour and for toning-in grey. The great advantage with semi-permanent colour is that because the colour can fade quickly it is ideal to experiment with – if you don't like the end result, simply wash it away. There will be no unsightly regrowth at the roots and because most semi-permanents have built-in conditioners your experiments will probably result in a lustrous head of hair which exudes vitality.

HIGH AND LOWS

Highlights and lowlights are by far the most popular forms of colouring hair. If you want to enhance your hair colour and make it shimmer and shine with subtle colour try lowlights. "One of my best male clients', says Sharon Dale, colourist, "had to tell his wife he'd had his hair low-lighted because it was so subtle she hadn't noticed. He was over the moon because those lowlights gave his confidence a discreet boost". Highlights are designed to lighten the hair and lowlights to tone in with it. The great thing about both techniques is that you can control how much or how little hair is coloured. The thicker the strands of treated hair, the more obvious the end result will be. Although regrowth does occur, it is barely visible as only odd strands of hair are affected.

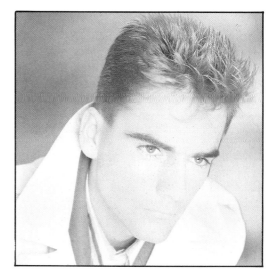

PERMANENT COLOURS

These take the form of tints and bleaches and are the only ones which can actually lighten hair. They work by penetrating the cuticle and entering the cortex, where the coloured molecules of the dye base combine with oxygen from the hydrogen peroxide in the product to make large molecules of dye. These become

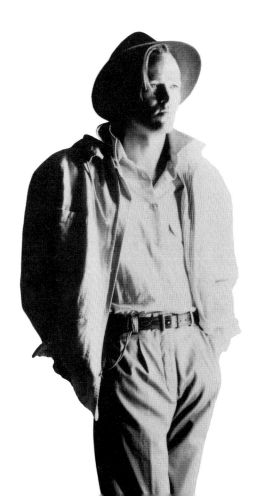

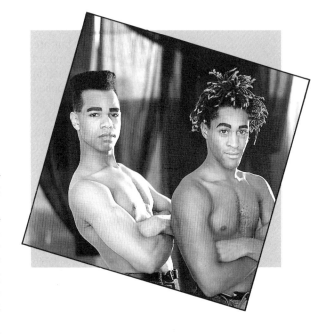

too large to pass back and are permanently locked within the cortex. The colour lasts just as long as the hair does which is why, if you want to retain the colour, roots have to be touched up as new hair grows. Because dark roots on a man look more obvious than they do on a woman, this could mean that you'll be returning to the salon as often as every two weeks!

There are several ways of highlighting and low-lighting hair. All involve selecting and colouring strands of hair. The hairdresser can use tinfoil, a cap, clingfilm or little, transparent plastic packets to separate the treated strands from the rest of the hair. Whatever method you opt for – and you should be given the choice – allow a couple of hours for this process. Selecting individual hair strands is painstaking and time consuming and the tint or bleach has to be left on for about 20 minutes to take effect.

The tinfoil method is the longest of all but it is kinder to the hair as it doesn't pull on it. Strands of hair are placed on squares of foil, the tint is applied with a brush and the hair is then wrapped in the foil. The clingfilm method works on a similar basis with the advantage that you and your colourist can see what is happening, how the process is "taking" and when the hair is ready. In recent years little plastic packets have been created which speed up this method as they are not so awkward to use as clingfilm can be. The cap, which is the speediest of them all as it involves no wrapping up of hair, resembles a swimming hat with little perforations. The cap is pulled down over the head, you can usually just peek out from under it, the strands of hair to be coloured are pulled through the perforations with a hook and the tint then applied. Because it is the quickest method it is also the cheapest but it can make the eyes smart and it puts pressure upon the hair as it is tugged through the cap.

COLOURING TECHNIQUES

Highlights and lowlights are only forerunners to many partial colouring techniques. Some of them disappear from the hair fashion frontier as quickly as they emerge but they do provide food for thought. Vidal Sassoon, for instance, have developed a technique especially for men called shoe-shine. The colour is applied to short hair on top of the head after it has been cropped, imparting a tinge of colour designed to reflect the natural shade and resulting in a glossy, polished appearance. Tortoise-shelling is ideal for brown heads of hair which can be complemented by hues of honeys, reds and hazels worked into the hair in alternation sections. A summery effect is achieved by touch-colouring, where just the ends of the hair are lightened. If you want your hair to shimmer with subtle colour, ask your stylist to apply tint on a vent brush and brush it through your hair.

If you've never tried colour before but are now yearning to have a go, don't be tempted into doing it at home. Even temporary wash-in colours can create an awful mess if applied single-handed and you really should consult an expert about the best shades for you. As a general rule you should never select a colour more than two shades lighter or darker than your natural shade, but rules are often broken. Some naturally dark men look sensational with cropped, bleached blond hair. Like choosing a style, hair colour depends to a great extent on your personality and the way you live. Make a subtle start with lowlights or a temporary rinse. Ask the hairdresser to show you a chart. It will contain swatches of hair with all the available colours on it which you can hold up to your own skin and hair to see how they blend.

Your colourist will probably want to perform a patch test and/or strand test before applying the colour. The patch test will make sure that your skin won't react badly to the chemicals she is about to use. A small amount of colour will be applied either at the back of the neck, behind the ear or in the inner elbow, and then left for 24 hours to give time for any possible reaction to erupt. Strand tests are often done by cutting off a small amount of hair and applying the colour to it to ensure that the chosen colour will work well on the hair. You can avoid this, however, by being totally honest about any colour you may have used on your hair in the past. Many salons have horror stories of hair turning green because a client has lied about the colours he or she has experimented with in the past!

Any good salon will try to sell you colour along with a new hair style. But another very good reason for seeking professional advice about how to colour your hair is that a hairdresser will tell you, in no uncertain terms, when not to colour. If your hair is not in good condition, if it has been damaged by too many perms or harsh treatment, then wait until new, healthier hair emerges. If you colour dry, damaged, porous hair, the cuticle will open rather than close, causing the colour to penetrate unevenly and resulting in a colour which is patchy and dull.

VEGETABLE DYES, AN ALTERNATIVE TREATMENT

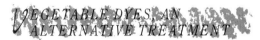

These were the earliest forms of hair colour – vegetable dyes were being used by the Egyptians 4000 years ago. They are substances obtained from various plants which, when suitably treated, can impart colour to human hair. Logwood and walnut skins are known to have been used for hair dyeing purposes, as have oak apples and rhubarb root, but the most common and effective vegetable dyes are camomile and henna.

Camomile is a plant which grows in Britain in the wild and in a cultivated state. It is particularly suitable for enhancing fair hair. There are various types of plant, but they look something like a large daisy, the heads of which can be collected and ground into a powder. This powder can be made into a paste, applied to the hair like a pack, left for about 15 minutes and then washed off. The resulting golden glint will vary in brightness depending on the hair's basic colour. A richer shade can always be obtained by leaving the dye on the hair for a longer period.

Henna is the powdered, dried leaves of the Egyptian privet (*Lawsonia Alba*) and is a dye for dark or auburn hair. It is applied in pack form much the same way as camomile and again has different effects according to the colour of your hair before use. Black hair will glisten with reddish tones and brown hair will take on a definite auburn hue.

> *Camomile can be used as a rinse to lighten fair hair. Simmer the dried flower heads with water and strain the resulting liquid. Pour over your hair after your normal shampoo and rinse to brighten your hair.*

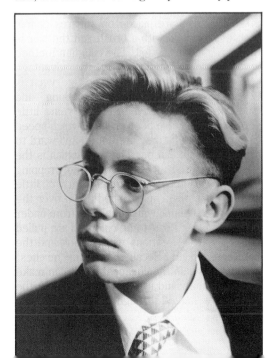

don't

Wash your hair in the bath. Hair is not properly washed if it is not rinsed thoroughly. Rinsing in bath water will not do, as the water will be dirty and full of scum and flakes of skin. Inadequate rinsing results in dull, lifeless hair and a flaking scalp.

Brush your hair when wet. It is far too fragile in this state to be treated so vigorously.

Be afraid to wash your hair as often as you think it needs it. If it's dirty, wash it every day if necessary.

Waste your money on expensive lotions and ointments if you are suffering from Male Pattern Baldness. They won't work. The situation is irreversible.

Let someone else buy your haircare products for you, they might be totally unsuitable for your type of hair.

do

Consult your hairdresser about which shampoos and conditioners you should be using. A good salon should be able to sell you some.

Take the trouble to find a salon and stylist that you like.

Communicate with your hairdresser. Tell him or her how you feel about your hair, what you dislike and like about it and how you would like it to look.

Comb through wet hair gently with a wide-toothed, saw cut comb.

do

Consult a trichologist if you are going bald and want to disguise the fact. he will inform you of the alternatives and advise you on where to go for help.

Eat a healthy, well balanced diet. Your hair is affected by what you eat. Gorge on chips and chocolate and your hair will become limp, dull and greasy. Balance out your food intake with fresh fruit and vegetables, lean meat, fish, poultry and fibre and your hair will exude health and vitality and so will you.

Learn to relax. Stress plays havoc with the hair as well as the heart. Take up a hobby, even if it's only reading for 20 minutes each day. It will help you to loosen up after the rigours of everyday life and reduce stress.

don't

Use very hot dryers on your hair; heat damages.

Panic if your hair seems to be falling out. Hair is constantly going through a growing, resting and shedding cycle and is bound to appear to be falling out some times. Some of us can lose up to 100 hairs per day but this is perfectly natural and there is no cause for concern.

Be afraid to say what you want, otherwise you'll be a dissatisfied customer for ever.

face

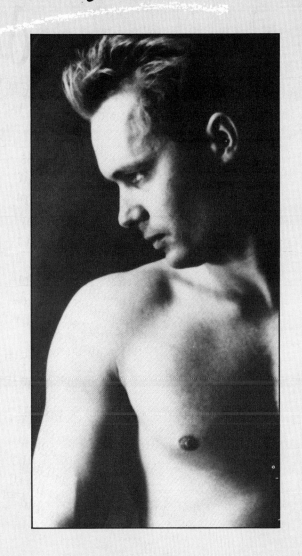

About face

When it comes to care and maintenance, a man and his face have not always been on the greatest terms. Traditionally they've met in the most uncongenial circumstances – first thing in the morning over a steamy bathroom mirror when the eyes are still half-glued with sleep and the mind's in a turmoil of pre-work rush and tear. Judging by the bare-toothed grimace he offers his reflected image whilst shaving against the clock, a man and his face might almost be at war.

Now no one suggests that a working guy treats his face to the daily equivalent of a candlelit dinner, but a little more informed thought (and where necessary, nurture) for what lies between the ears, would, as young men are now increasingly aware, not come amiss.

A BIGGER SPLASH

The generation that's now reached elder statesman and grandaddy status made its own breakthrough with the realization that aroma of Old Spice was far more appealing than odour of Old Sock. Over the last five years another quantum leap has been achieved: the men's toiletry business has more than doubled and is still growing at some 20 per cent a year. Market researchers are murmuring of a male beauty revolution with £215 million a year being spent on men's brands in the UK – mostly in chemists, but increasingly in department stores. Aftershaves and colognes (which men will still splash on their cheeks instead of their bodies) are major sellers. Ever-new brand names appear on the shopping shelves, each carefully targeted at a particular male species: the traditional, the athletic, the romantic, the post-punk – or the pure peacock. Although the average man spends no more than £11 a year on toiletries, single men and those under 25 spend nearly double, and will think nothing of splashing out £20 on a single bottle of the fragrance favoured by a girlfriend. Enlightened – or perhaps merely mean – males are also borrowing from their girlfriends.

CUT THROAT COMPETITION

Across in the shaving industry, a battle of the razor rages: In recent years throwaway plastic gizmos from Bic, Gillette and Wilkinson have proved an enormous hit with the young – cheap, brightly designed and as easily portable as your overnight toothbrush. But now the electric element is fighting back. Wet-shave, dry shave or a quick battery workover driving to work, one thing's for sure: the force – the competitive market force – is very much with you, and pulling out. The days when Desperate Dan (he of the *Dandy* comic) was obliged to bash his wiry whiskers back in with a hammer are gone for good.

FACE MANUAL

It's also possible that the days of self-deceiving macho doublethink are numbered: by some curious quirk of masculine logic it's always been not only acceptable but a positive source of pride to own a well-serviced car – but a well-serviced face – well that smacks uncomfortably of camp. You read your motor manual from cover to cover, and you don't expect your "wheels" to run really well unless regularly topped up with petrol and fresh oil. Isn't it a little perverse to tend to a Ferrari or a Fiat, yet expect your physiognomy to take care of itself?

FACING THE PAST

In the past certainly it's taken more than a streak of extrovert bravado to admit to self-pampering. Only a powerful character like the Sun King, Louis XIV, would perform an extravagant toilette in front of an invited audience. It took the ultimate Regency dandy, Beau Brummell, to make it known that he required a good two hours to clean his teeth, shave and attend to his eyebrows and whiskers with tweezers and an enlarging mirror before even beginning to dress. But the Beau's attitude to grooming was not just a puff of precious powder: "There is", he reasonably observed, "as much vanity and coxcombry in slovenliness as in its most extravagant opposite."

BALANCING ACT

What's needed, as the circus ringmaster told the high-wire walker, is balance. Without going OTT on the eyebrow plucking à la Boy George, or falling prey to the romantic self-worship of Dorian Gray, you can still aim to put your best face forward.

Your face, after all, is your number one feature, the visible source of your expression and individual identity. Time may modify that first impression, but social psychologists say you can't stop people drawing instant inferences from your fizzog in less time than it takes to make an introduction: if you wear spectacles, the chances are you're taken for intelligent; a leathery skin for some reason suggests hostility, thick lips are seen as sexy, thin lips as diligent. A depressive person may have his attitude written all over his countenance – jowls of slouching apathy, while a cheerful chap has laugh lines to prove it. Evidence that men, at least as much as women, are judged by the countenance they keep, lies in the popular application of 'physical landmarks' nicknames: Ol' Blue Eyes, Piranha Teeth, Nosey, Pug and Parrot Face to name but a few.

It's therefore well worth thinking a bit about this face of yours, the flagship of your figure. You wouldn't set about stripping down your car engine without first enquiring 'How To'. Why then have so many men been happy to scrape away at their faces with as much skill as if they were taking a Brillo pad to a frying pan?

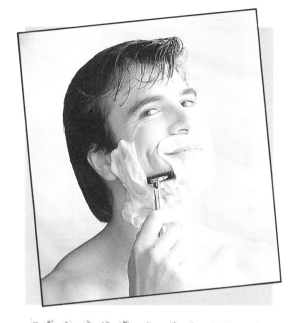

LOOKS NATURAL

But what's really liberating about looks today is that you no longer have to be a clone of a current idol. The old image of the male model as 'Wimpo' man has given way to a dozen assorted styles. As one international model agency put it: "Our men are terribly different, yet all do well. We've one who was discovered on a building site and who works out for four hours a day. We've another who's totally non-muscular, very much the English eccentric type, with receding hair and furrowed brow. He works every day and is in such demand we could book him twice over."

It's not which look that matters so much as the degree of fresh grooming that goes with it. You can't advertise your face in *Exchange and Mart*, or trade it in for a new model as if it were a Fiat or a Ferrari, so don't treat it thus. Give it due care and maintenance and it will give you lasting, all-weather service.

F
A
C
E

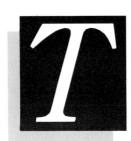

The close shave

Removal men: the statistics

A man's face has anything between 6000–25,000 hairs: some 800 per square inch on the chin, and only 250 on the lower cheek. Like a porcupine's back, these hairs are graduated in scale from a bristly .008 inch thickness on the chin to a finer .002 close to the sideboards.

The vast majority of men (some 93 per cent) take 'em off daily, using up an average three minutes each morning, which over a lifetime represents six months dedicated to the razor regime. Most men claim to find the business of dispensing with 27 and a half feet of living whisker (55 years' estimated profusion) an unremitting chore. Yet paradoxically a survey has revealed that 97 per cent of men decided they would not use a product to remove facial hair permanently even if such a magic potion were invented.

The beard is plainly bound up with strong psychological sentiments. Its first growth, after all, is the acceptable face, if you like, of male sexuality. Perhaps subconsciously too, men recognize that the way their beard grows can also be a weathervane for their condition. Stress, tension and anxiety can speed up growth of beard (all that adrenalin coursing through the veins), while alcohol abuse slows it down.

Every man has experienced mornings when for no particular reason he cuts himself once whilst shaving. In general the aggressive, impatient chap at odds with himself and the world is more likely to hack away at his face in a daily scrape that's like ploughing up hardcore, than the man at peace with his world who takes time and trouble to prepare his skin for a smooth remove.

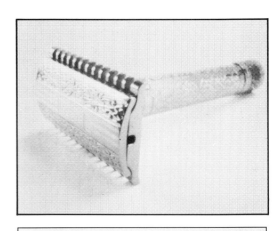

21 million men shave in the UK today. In 1986 they spent an estimated £53 million on shaving gear – materials to make the rough going smooth. They bought some 490 million razor blades.

Wet shave, sir . . . or dry?

Roughly 60 per cent – or two out of three men – are wet or mechanical shavers, 33 per cent opt for the dry (or electric) method, the rest of course being non-shaving beardies. From time to time men cross the great divide and change their method. A good number own both razor and electric shaver, ringing the changes depending upon their mood and the time available. But if you've always been a dry shaver who fancies splashing out, do make the change gradually. Introduce wet shaving once a week at first and build up gradually, or your skin could suffer soreness, rashes and general shellshock.

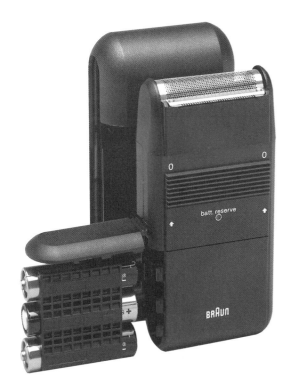

WATER WORKS

As every professional will tell you, water works. Kenneth Grange is a leading designer of both razors and shavers. He believes that more men who wet shave enjoy the process. Rather than viewing it as an evil necessity they see it as an essentially agreeable, serious celebration of water and time and cleanliness. Dry shaving, says Grange, is by contrast essentially a massaging process: "You can often tell a dry shavee because he has one stray long hair sticking out because after a day or two missing it, the blades on his electric shaver aren't designed to pick it up."

However good the high speed blade on your modern electric there's a tendency for it to rip rather than cut the face, leaving behind a ragged surface. Usually too, it's very hard to achieve a really close shave because the razor is cutting a foil's thickness from your face. Dry shavers will probably notice the dreaded 'five o'clock shadow' earlier in the evening than their wet razor brothers. Wet shavers often have a more lively glow about their faces, because their style of shaving is a very good exfoliator, removing the dead skin cells that look dull and flaky. But there's also a danger when wet shaving of taking off living skin cells too by overdoing the close shave – that's when you can feel sore and sensitive.

Shaving can be good for your looks in ways you least suspect – experts say that the facial contortions involved tone and exercise your muscles – keeping you in sleek cheek shape longer.

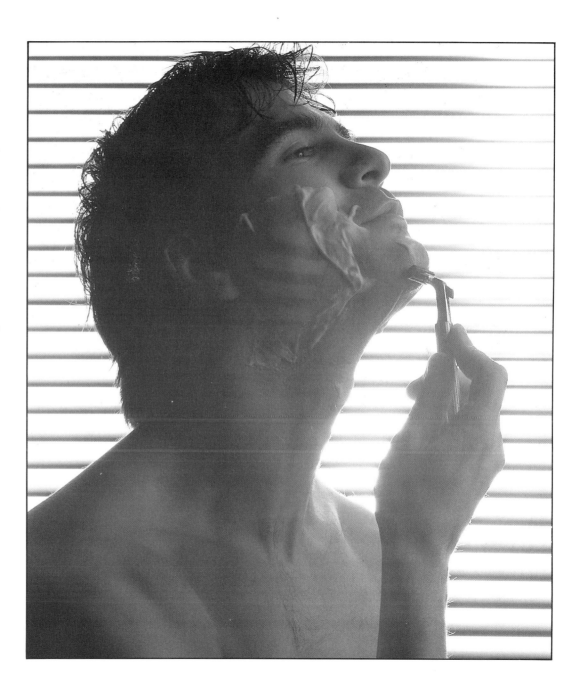

**F
A
C
E**

WHICH WET RAZOR – ARE YOU CONFUSED, OR SPOILED FOR CHOICE?

It's curious that men who are supposed to be the enquiring, adventurous sex frequently use the razor they saw their father use. Kenneth Graham inherited several cuthroats which his father had used for years and years – and he still resorts to them now and again "because I enjoy the extraordinary dexterity needed to do the job well."

Real men, so the rumour goes, are rather keen on a cuthroat comeback. Kenneth Grange says the cuthroat razor definitely gives the closest of all shaves and though it does require greater skill, he "doesn't mind the bloodletting as long as there's a styptic pencil to staunch the flow." The styptic pencil acts as a blood clotting agent, just moisten the tip and apply. Don't attempt to mop up with cotton wool unless you want to look like a parody of Old Father William.

JAWBONE JUNGLE

Beyond the good old cuthroat the market branches into a sophisticated, very fast-changing and sometimes bewildering jungle of options. Those who haven't taken Dad's brand on board will choose, perhaps only half consciously, according to weight, balance, packaging and general look and feel of the product. But how many men have totally mastered the subtle difference between a twin-bladed razor with fixed head as opposed to its swivel head counterpart? Or does blind brand loyalty prevail? As for sending your lady out to buy on your behalf, unless you specifically direct her she'll have a hell of a job choosing for you. Ten to one the fur would fly before you'd even opened the packet.

Here's a breakdown of the wet razor types currently on offer:

THE DOUBLE-EDGED This is the good old traditional model of which the original Gillette Safety Razor was grandaddy. Some 12 per cent of wet shavers choose these, and they're generally regarded as the serious operators. Basically these razors have sturdy macho handles, often in metal, which takes a flat blade sharpened at both ends so you can use either side as you manoeuvre round facial contours. Classic examples are the Gillette and the Wilkinson Sword Classic.

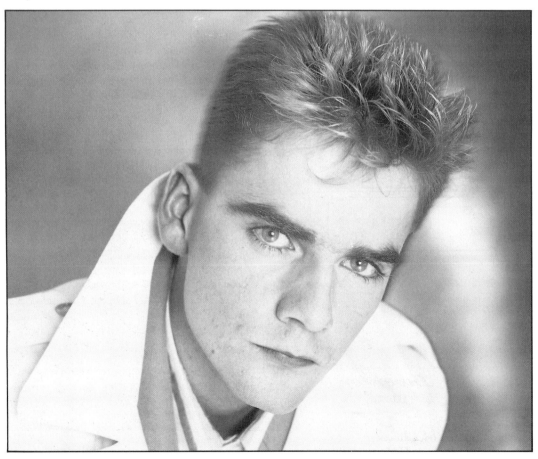

The styptic pencil is made of granular ammonia aluminium sulphate and iron-free aluminium sulphate.

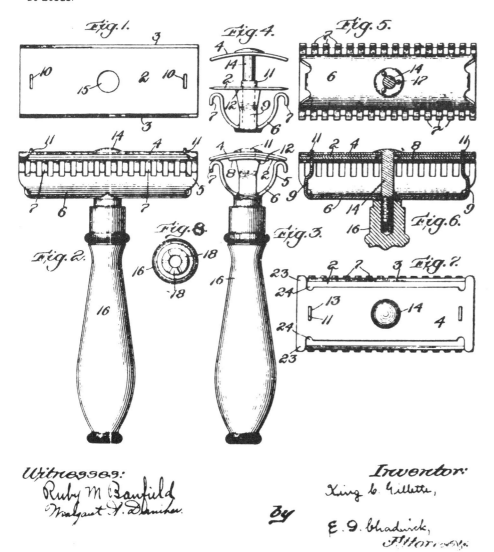

No. 775,134. PATENTED NOV. 15, 1904.

K. C. GILLETTE.
RAZOR.
APPLICATION FILED DEC. 3, 1901.

NO MODEL.

Fig. 1.

Fig. 4.

Fig. 5.

Fig. 2.

Fig. 8.

Fig. 3.

Fig. 6.

Fig. 7.

Witnesses:
Ruby M Banfield
Margaret A Danaher

Inventor:
King C. Gillette,
By
E. D. Chadwick,
Attorney.

THE SYSTEMS RAZOR Increasingly popular with about 22 per cent of the wet shave market share. With a permanent handle either metal or plastic, the systems razor has a totally disposable clip-on blade unit which can be picked up automatically without you're touching it – an added safety and convenience factor. Systems razors use twin blades for a particularly close shave: the geometry of these blades is such that every hair is cut twice. What actually happens when a strand of hair is shaved is a process known in the trade as hysterisis. The skin stretches and the individual hair pulls further out of the follicle for a moment before sinking back. The twin blade action means it is cut again just before retracting and when its greatest length is exposed. Popular systems razors are the Kenneth Graham Profile for Wilkinson Sword and the Gillette Contour Plus. The Gillette Contour Plus also features a patent Lubrastrip – a water-soluble lubricant designed to make a close shave more gentle.

DISPOSABLES Only arrived on the scene in the mid 1970s. Although they're absolutely without owner appeal, disposables are now positively grabbing the market with a 68 per cent hold on wet shavers. They're extraordinarily low-cost, ideal for travelling and as a hasty 'distress purchase' for anyone suddenly finding themselves away from home for a night. Gillette, Wilkinson Sword and Bic lead the market.

SWIVEL OR FIXED Just to complicate matters still more systems razors and disposables are made with a choice of fixed heads or swivel, which are intended to adapt to the individual face contours with greater ease. The Gillette Contour and the Wilkinson Sword Profile with swivel action are probably the best all-purpose wet razors for anyone who finds the process at all difficult.

FACE

YOURS TRULY

A razor is a very personal object and should never be shared – even among members of one family. The government AIDS information leaflet warns specifically against sharing shaving kit with anyone suspected of having AIDS or carrying the HIV virus.

Rinse your used razor thoroughly and shake off excess water. Do not dry the blade or handle it unnecessarily or you could damage its edge. Store in a clean dry condition – and never place in boiling water.

Dropping or knocking it could affect its alignment – handle with as much care as you use it!

WET SHAVING – THE PERFECT PERFORMANCE

Judging by the way many men go about it you could think there was nothing more scientific to the daily shave than slicing the top off a boiled egg. But it's surprising how few men have thought or can articulate the hows and wherefores of the process. Most say they just picked the craft up as they went along, or had it straight from Dad's chin. One otherwise well groomed editor of a London weekly confessed that after years he'd only just twigged you were meant to shave downwards instead of up – and he was finding it hard to kick the habit!

The Bic disposable razor (first in the market) represents another succès fou for the rich, reclusive plastics entrepreneur Baron Biche of France, whose two previous smash-hit selling products are the ubiquitous see-through Biro and the chuckaway lighter.

Here's how

Warmth as well as wetness is a Good Shave factor – keep your bathroom heated if you can. Professionals give the hot towel treatment – try squeezing out your own very hot, wet flannel and placing it on your face for a moment. Make sure it's quite dry – hot water could burn you whereas steam opens your pores and prepares your face for shaving. Shaving under the steamy shower is also a good idea.

First wash your face – with soap and warm water. Don't make the water too hot or your face may swell. Rinse before applying shaving cream, stick, soap or foam. French figures suggest that of the 37 per cent of men who use a shaving brush, four per cent also use a stick, 12 per cent something out of a pot and 21 per cent shaving foam. Of the rest 51 per cent use aerosol shaving foam; three per cent shaving cream and nine per cent nothing – or plain soap.

A rush job could be a second-rate job. If you shave as soon as you wake, your face will still be puffy from sleep, and the muscles relaxed. If you can, wait about 30 minutes after getting up by which time that 'melting mask' will have pulled itself together. Your muscles will have toned up, pushing out the bristles of your beard. If you shave before this you could well notice a shadow creeping back by mid-morning.

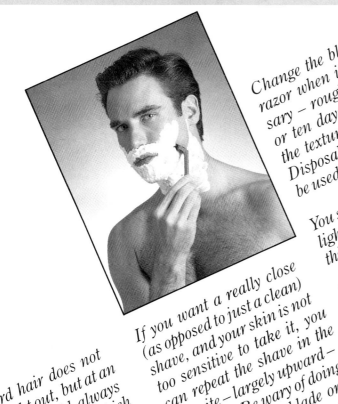

Change the blade on your razor when it seems necessary – roughly once a week or ten days, depending on the texture of your beard. Disposables can generally be used for about five days.

You should shave with short, light strokes and rinse every third stroke or so.

Finish with a splash of cold water to close the pores and prevent dust and dirt getting in.

If you want a really close shave, and your skin is not too sensitive to take it, you can repeat the shave in the opposite – largely upward – direction. Be wary of doing this with a new blade or if your skin is not used to wet shaving. (as opposed to just a clean)

Your beard hair does not grow straight out, but at an angle. You should always shave with the grain, which usually means shaving downwards, starting at the hair junction by the ear. Shaving the wrong way could cause ingrown hairs which are sore and painful. Shaving underneath the chin your razor should travel from front to back. The growth angle on the neck means that most men will shave this hair with upwards stroke.

Skin sabbatical: If you can, rest your face from shaving once a week: the shave you get after a 48 hour break is particularly good.

As for acne or simple pimples, wet shaving will do them no harm provided your face is clean before you start. Dry shaving is not so healthy for spots as you could spread infection and grow a whole new crop with a waterless shave.

Well done, a shave should be invigorating and set you up for the day, feeling freshly groomed.

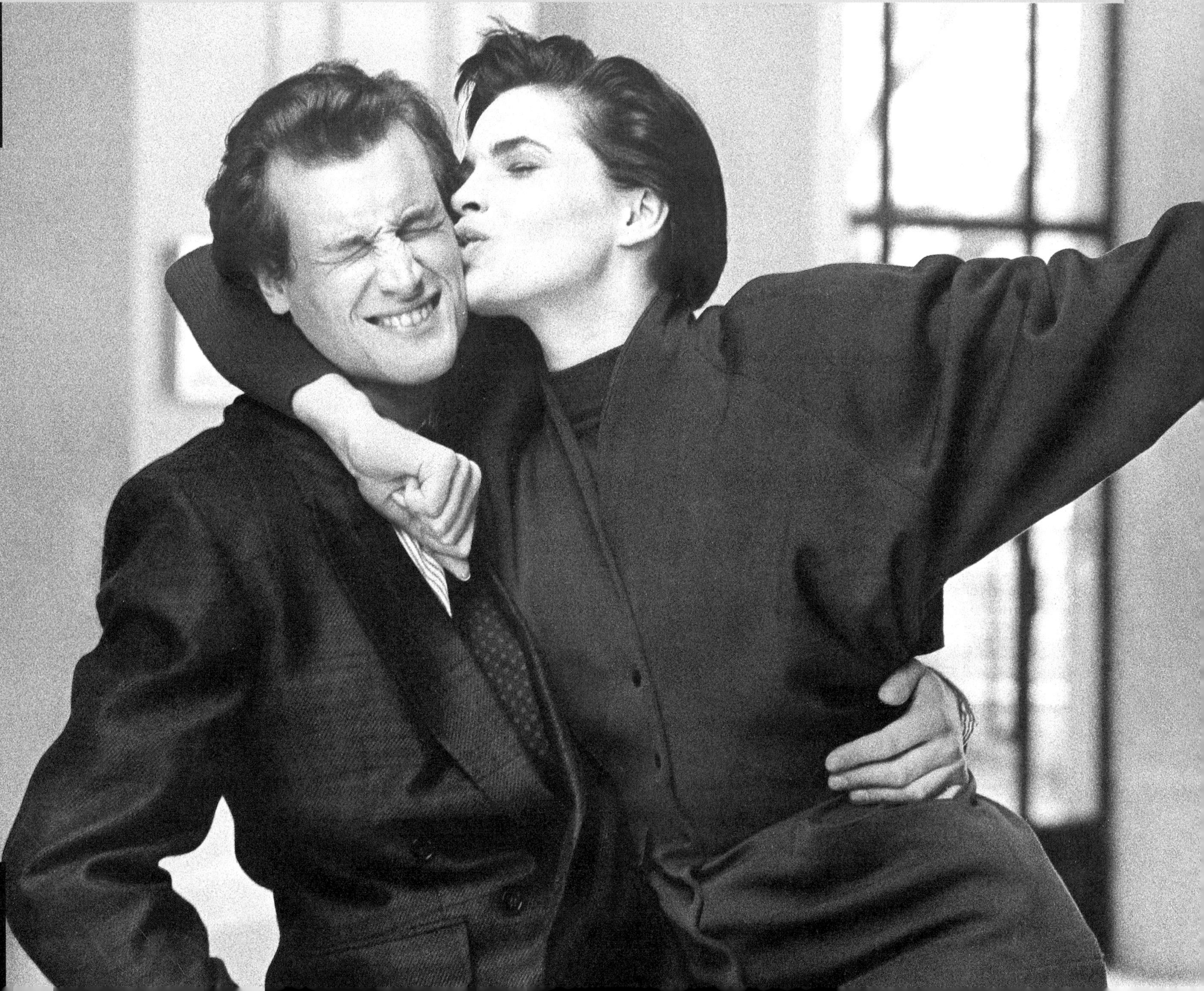

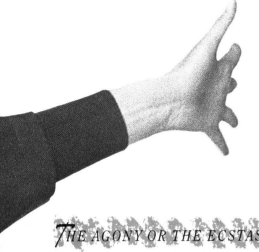

THE AGONY OR THE ECSTASY?

You may want to alleviate the dry tautness of a new-shaven face, but you certainly don't have to suffer aftershave agony. It's not so much machism-atic, as madly masochistic to splash alcohol-filled aftershave on sore or cut skin. You might as well put surgical spirit on an open wound. Some men do enjoy the light tingle of aftershave, but try instead one of the many soothing moisturizing skin balms now on the market just for the purpose. New Zealand-born John Field, who developed Skin Fitness after a lifetime's experience in the cosmetic industry, is particularly adamant that "no man wants a shiny face. He may not really even like the slightly feminine association of the word 'moisturizer.' But there's nothing more suitable to describe what he does want – something to put back in his skin what shaving's taken out."

ARE YOU BEING BADGERED?

The badger shaving brush, as all the best badgers tell you, has no equal as a water carrier from basin to face. The House of Kent, leading British brush-makers since 1777 (and holders of the Royal Warrant), explain that badger brushes are pricey (from about £10 to £200 or £300 for a really fine example set in gold or ivory handle – such as one recently made for presentation to the King of Jordan). They are costly because the making process is painstaking, skilled and largely hand-crafted. You could also use second quality badger, or a badger bristle mix – or even, if you've a very stiff beard, pure bristle. Beware imitations – some cheap brushes have the hair dyed to fake the real thing.

After use the badger brush should be hung upside down to drain and dry naturally. Well looked after, a good brush should last ten, twelve or even fifteen years – if it's not been rubbed too hard, too often.

But . . . and it's a major but, anyone who is anything of an animal lover will probably prefer to buy imitation to the real badger thing. British badgers are a safely protected species, so badger hair has to be imported either from China or from the Pyrenees, where the silver-tipped badger is hunted in the wild expressly for its hair. The RSPCA recommend avoiding use of any product which has involved killing or otherwise causing an animal suffering. Any of the 84 Body Shops now in the UK should be able to supply you with a synthetic bristle brush with the hair dyed in bright fun colours.

Aerosol application of course requires no brush. And what, wonders John Field of Skin Fitness, is wrong with your hand as a means of applying water, soap or cream anyway? Fingers, to borrow old Nanny's dictum about forks, were made before brushes.

MOUSSE-TIQUE

The aerosol foam lobby is definitely growing – it's had 2.6 million converts in the last ten years according to one French survey. But it seems a switch could be on the way and that cream may now be returning as the *crème de la crème* of shaving preparations. Aerosol, it's now being said, stands off the skin which is not terribly useful to your shave, albeit lubricating. Cream, however, encompasses each bristle at the base, reducing razor drag and making the shave smoother.

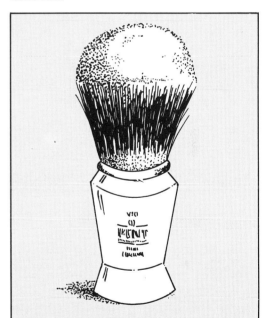

Pure badger hair taken from the animal's back is the best available quality. It should have very white tips and a very black stripe in the middle. The stronger the contrast, the better the quality.

HOME AND DRY SHAVING

If ease and a consistent shave are priorities then you must invest in a shaver. If you're a novice shaver, don't be fobbed off with Dad's ancient appliance unserviced for years. Start the way you mean to go on, selecting your shaver from the various options of battery, mains, rechargeable and rechargeable and mains. It's worth making the right choice from the word go because 85 per cent of users stay loyal to the same brand when replacing their shaver.

Battery operated shavers are the most economic and they're handy – but really only suitable for occasional use. But the best option is an elegant shaver that's both mains and rechargeable which has been designed especially for young shavers under 24 who buy 42 per cent of all shavers sold.

COMPETITIVE CUT THRUST AND FOIL

In the shaver market the main division lies between the rotary system and the foil system. There is also a triple-action slot-head system for those who shave rigorously and might find foil shavers too sensitive. Experts agree that the foil systems give a closer shave than the rotary, although Philips rotary shavers are definitely beloved by a more conservative sector of the market. For those who like to hedge their bets the Japanese (Panasonic) have come up with a wet and dry shaver. The rechargeable shaver can be used dry or with foam, or even under the shower.

FAULTS FOILED

Just how much servicing your electric shaver needs depends not only on the make, but on the grain of your beard, your personal attitude to mechanical upkeep – and good luck.

One man claims to have used his Remington shaver for 30 years without once having it overhauled; others, say Remington, send theirs off for a check-up as soon as the motor pitch sounds a little out of the ordinary. Some people expect to live and die with the shaver inherited from their fathers; others positively enjoy trading in for a new model every three years. Philips say their shavers need only be sent for servicing when something is obviously wrong. Braun recommend a professional clean-and-cosset every eighteen months.

Before buying it's worth checking out just how much regular home maintenance each individual manufacturer recommends. Also, check how many service agents the manufacturer recommends – and if there's one near your home.

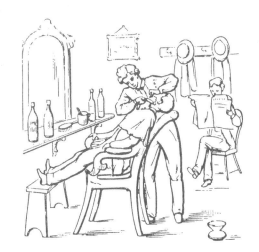

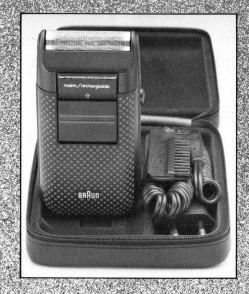

DRY RUN – HOW TO GET THE BEST DRY SHAVE

Apply, if you wish, your chosen pre-electric shave.

Dry the skin very well.

Apply your shaver without pressing too hard, stretching the skin a little for best results.

Lastly, apply an aftershave balm.

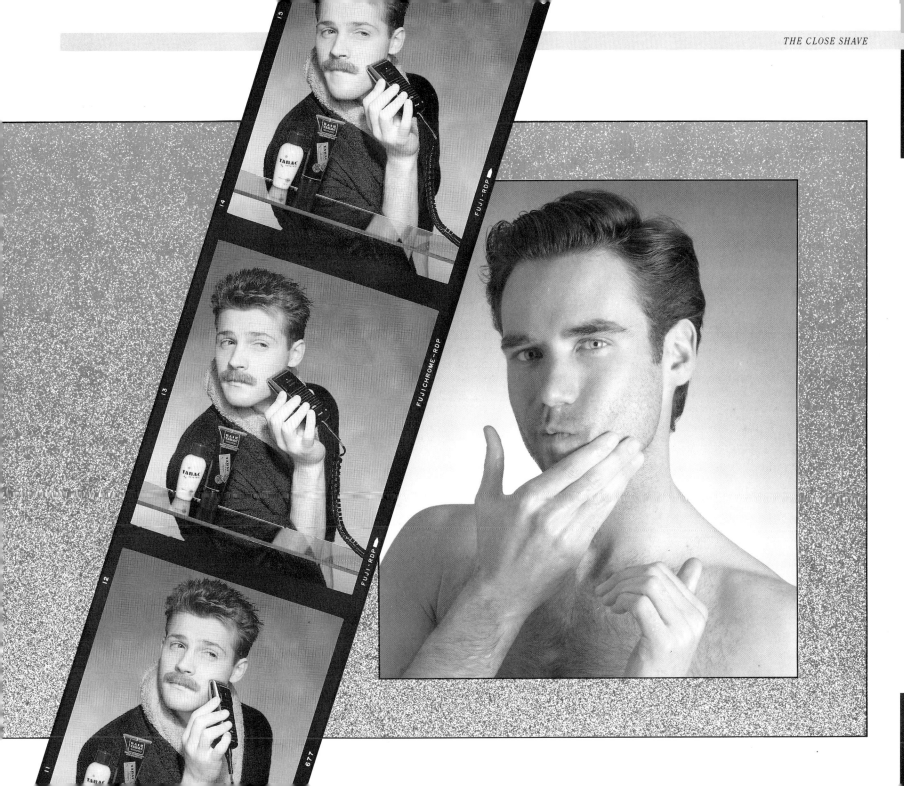

COMING UP TRUMPERS

As more and more hairdressers go unisex, and the old barber's shops with the striped poles outside disappear, fewer and fewer master barbers remain. If you have one who shaves professionally in your home town, or know a little man in the City, for heaven's sake cultivate and frequent this dying species. It's a rare and relaxing experience having the open razor and hot towel treatment.

Trumper of Curzon Street, London, offer the ultimate gentleman's shave in their celebrated olde-worlde premises. Here be mahogany booths, marble washstands and huge crystal decanters full of their own shampoos and fragrances, alongside displays of the most covetable shaving equipment and quality brushes.

Mr Lenard has been shaving gentlemen since he was 14 and has been with Trumpers itself for 41 years – during which he's often dropped parcels of goodies off at the Palace. Mr Lenard remembers the days when a gentleman would come in for his shave every day "but now only a few regulars – mostly businessmen come in most days. For the majority of clients it's a special occasion treat, being shaved – and we do have some men who come in on their wedding day for fear they'll be too nervous to do it themselves without botching the job!"

Mr Lenard is the absolute antithesis of the dread old Sweeney Todd demon barber who felled his unsuspecting customers with one cutthroat stroke and dispatched them to the basement below via a trap door. Mr Lenard is a soothing, benevolent out-and-out professional, solicitous in his white coat – his number one interest to relax and unwind his clients. "The idea is that a man should feel completely relaxed before I start. To this end I squeeze out a really hot flannel very well – so it's still steaming but quite dry. This I lay on his face. Warm water cotton wool pads go over his eyes for a minute or two while I get my materials ready. Then it's a first-class shave finished off with talcum all over the face and cotton wool dipped in a fragrance like our own Extract of Limes. You know the client's enjoyed it when he stands up, draws himself in and sucks his lips and cheeks in. The look on his face is the best response I can have." It takes about 15 to 20 minutes.

Trumper's also do a face massage with vanishing cream, hot towels – and cold water to finish. "When it's over" promises Mr Lenard "the skin feels new and you feel rejuvenated."

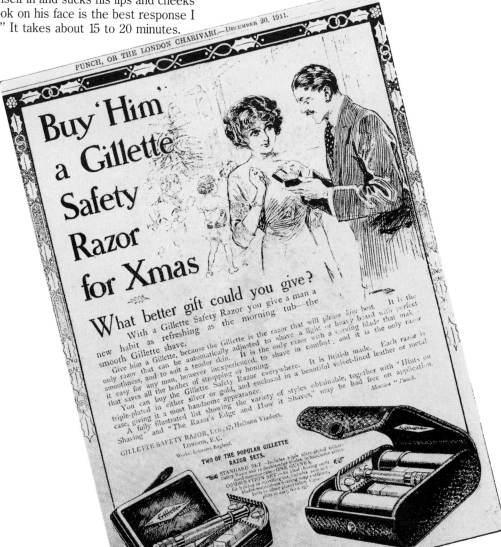

CIVILIZATION IS FOR SMOOTHIES

Since man is constantly trying to improve upon Nature, you could argue that the urge to shave is just another manifestation of his ongoing efforts. Efforts that go back four million years, say archaeologists who've unearthed the earliest shaving implements in hard metal from ancient Egyptian and Babylonian earthworks.

Whether to shave or not has always proved a bit of a conflict. Although it's been considered manly to be hairy, it's also by some strange paradox considered more civilized, more hygienic, even more holy to take off the facial hair. Egyptian high priests for instance shaved all over face and body, but their Pharaohs reflected the ultimate paradox of the shaving issue – they took off their real beards, presumably to prove they were gentlemen of great refinement, then put on long thin false beards to symbolize their power and rank.

But how to take the beard off? That was ever the question.

ROMAN RAVAGES Resourceful Romans developed an early depilatory which to modern ears sounds dreadful: they smeared their faces with an unguent called *dropacista*, largely made up of pitch and resin, but reinforced for extra efficacy by ivy gum, ass's fat, goat's gall, bat's blood or ashes of snake. And to think we sometimes view it as masochistic to slap astringent aftershave on a gentle face of today! Still, *dropacista* was apparently good enough for Julius Caesar.

The alternative was to visit the 'tonsor', whose dodgy utensils included iron razors sharpened on special Spanish stone and applied straight to the unprepared, unlubricated skin surface. Ouch! Cuts and grazes were so common that the authorities laid fines per wound inflicted by these barber-torturers.

Pliny the Elder, the natural historian, cooked up an aftershave balm of his own: spiders' webs soaked in oil and vinegar. His motto? 'Fortune favours the brave'.

DO IT YOURSELF Clean shaven men of the Middle Ages were only as smooth as their barber made them. Even in 1664 Samuel Pepys, the great diarist, obviously thought he'd stumbled on the best DIY invention yet when he "began a practice which I find by the ease I do it with, that I shall continue, it saving me money and time, that is to trimme myself with a razor – which pleases me mightily".

A WHIM FOR THE WHISKER In 1762 the first mechanical razor with hooded lid was invented by a French master-tailor, Jean-Jacques Perret. A similar, improved steel-bladed model was produced in Sheffield in the 1820s.

HAIL, KING GILLETTE!

The great modern safety razor we owe to a Canadian-born travelling salesman, King Camp Gillette. King Gillette passed a number of frustrated years trying to conjure-up some everyday object that would transform his fortunes. Early morning irritation with his own blunt razor one day brought home to King that he held the answer in his hands.

In 1903, his company's first year in production, 51 razor sets and 168 blades were sold. By 1905 sales figures had risen to 250,000 razors and two million blades. During the First World War the US Government placed an order with Gillette to kit out the entire US armed forces going to Europe – three and a half million razors and 36 million blades!

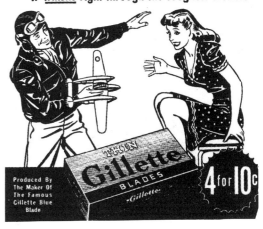

A real <u>long</u>-<u>lasting</u> low-priced blade
Is Thin Gillette—the finest made!
Slick, speedy shaves are now no trouble...
It <u>whisks</u> right through the toughest stubble!

Produced By The Maker Of The Famous Gillette Blue Blade

THIN Gillette BLADES *Gillette*

4 for 10c

"The Gillette Safety Razor Company has practically revolutionized a whole industry and the act of shaving as well, and to some degree has changed the habits of mankind. There is no other article for individual use so universally known or widely distributed. In my travels I have found it in the most northern town of Norway and in the Sahara desert."

King Camp Gillette

In Boston, USA the Gillette Shaving Research Centre has 22 laboratories where 300 employees shave for a living – being monitored as they put blade to face at different times of the day.

Keep your hair on

BEARDS AND MOUSTACHES

According to recent research, only seven per cent of British men resist the daily shave. 93 per cent of women, we're told, prefer them without a whisker. This is no modern revelation: "Lord" shudders Beatrice in Shakespeare's *Much Ado About Nothing*, "I could not endure a husband with a beard on his face".

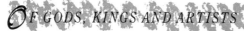

OF GODS, KINGS AND ARTISTS

The beard has been subject to the ebbs and flows of fashion. In ancient Greece beards were associated with wisdom and maturity. Dignitaries and philosophers, notably Socrates, wore them and senior gods such as Jupiter were depicted in statue bearded.

British beards flourished in periods of fierce patriotism. Stout-hearted Britons refused to abandon theirs despite pressure from conquering Romans to shave and be civilized. Under the great queens Elizabeth I and Victoria beards proved particularly popular.

The advent of the 17th century perruke put wigs before whiskers for almost two centuries, but early in the 19th century the beard was back as a defiant symbol of revolutionary politics. Lord Byron's subtle arrangement for lip and chin during his Albanian-gothic phase gave facial hair a dash of romance.

Royalty in the portly personage of Edward VII gave the beard a fine fillip but by the 1920s they were reduced to features of fun. In the early Fifties it was rare enough to meet a bearded man on a small town street to excite comment. But beards crept back with the beat generation and have remained with us ever since, though still more popular with certain professions than with others. Among archaeologists, sailors, inventors, musicians and theatrical gentlemen, the beard denotes non-conformity, creativity and a sense of spirit and adventure.

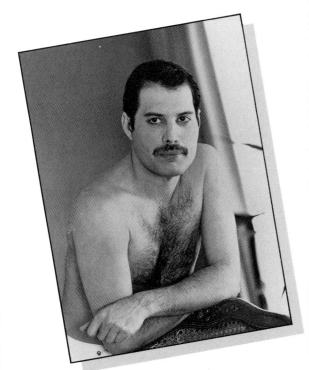

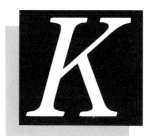

Egyptian queens, as well as kings, were portrayed as bearded to signify their status.

FIT FOR THE JOB

But are beards businesslike? Not long ago a salesman applying for a job with a multi-national computer monolith was told he'd only be hired on condition he did violence to his facial fuzz. He agreed – but only on condition that they first offered him the job. . . . Are beards suitably royal? Prince Michael of Kent obviously believes so, but the Queen Mother has grave doubts: "I told him quite frankly that I didn't like it at all", she pronounced of Prince Charles' short-lived barbarity.

The average man has about 15,500 beard hairs on his face which grow at the rate of three and three quarter millimetres each day or five and a half inches per year.

Young Romans dedicated the shorn hair from their first beards to Apollo or Venus as a token of gratitude for reaching manhood and to propitiate the now useful Goddess of Love.

Alexander the Great had his men shave before the Battle of Arbela in 331 BC to prevent the enemy from seizing or 'bearding' them by the chin.

In AD 117 the Emperor Hadrian decided to grow a beard as a disguise for his battle scars.

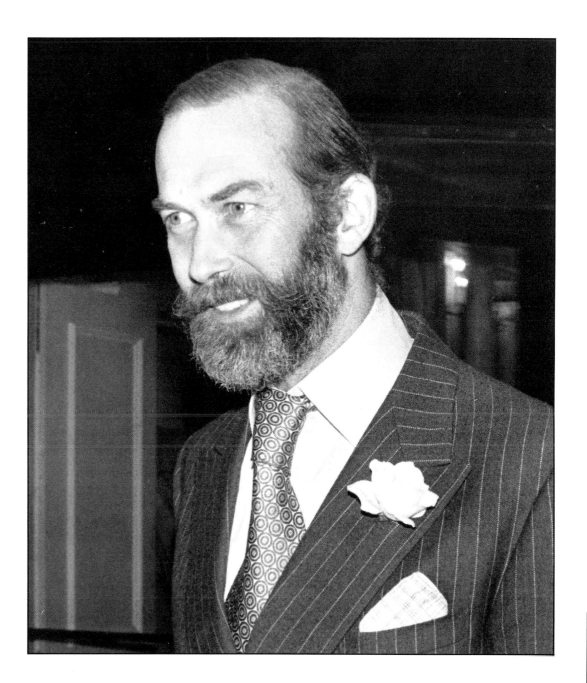

FACE

STARTING FROM SCRATCH

Who in creation's the gent best-placed to grow a beard from scratch? Why Robinson Crusoe of course. The perfect excuse (his shaving tackle had gone overboard) was enhanced by his enforced isolation (no one to rib him as he passed through the five days to a week stage of growth when the Tender Plant upon one's chin lends its owner strong similarity to a Parkhurst prison escapee). Crusoe also had plenty else (including the small matter of finding food and shelter) to divert him from rushing to a rock pool every five minutes to see how much longer the whiskers had waxed.

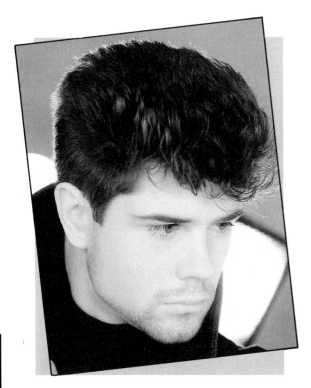

A WATCHED BEARD NEVER GROWS Just as a watched pot never boils, so a beard subjected to excess scrutiny will never progress fast enough to satisfy and consequently is likely to end up down the plughole. If you're serious about the whole hairy business you must be patient – and also intelligent about the time and place when the inevitably unprepossessing stages of your burgeoning beard can be got through unremarked. It is obviously foolish to attempt facial hair growth shortly before:

1. Your wedding.
2. An important job interview.
3. Having your photograph taken as a permanent record of public or private achievement (unless you're a megastar, see entry on designer stubble).
4. A court appearance (do you want the Judicial Presence to prejudge you as a recidivist, or at least as one who doesn't care enough for authority to use a razor?)
5. Travelling to a far-flung or politically sensitive country for which an entry visa has been obtained after considerable effort accompanied by passport photos in triplicate which depict you as unequivocally cleanshaven.

Some men start growing beards during a bout of 'flu on the grounds that "since I'm too weak to hold a razor I may as well get feeling awful and looking frightful over in one fell swoop." Others choose summer holiday time: all very well if you don't suffer from heat sensitivity, which a burgeoning beard on sore skin may well aggravate. It is also useful to have the Greek or the Espagnol to explain "This moulting privet hedge appearance is strictly temporary. Soon I shall resemble the fine film producer David Puttnam." Without the lingo – forget it. No holiday romance was ever encouraged by dancing cheek to cheek with sandpaper. If you must persist be quite sure you won't get cold feet about your furry face and shave the lot off before returning to the office.

But do check out the office culture first: today, at last, most straight-laced multi-national companies do permit beards – even fairly scraggy undergrowth, it's reported from one city office. But Yuppy accountants in the larger double-barrelled name companies, barristers and bankers, may still find bosses too conservative to risk a face on their clients that looks to have been lately dipped in ash.

> *Persian kings had gold thread woven into their beards as a sign of wealth and status.*

> _Vain King Louis XIV shaved off his beard at 42 when he first found white hairs in it._

> _Only in the 1850s did the British Army lift its anti-beard regulations so that soldiers serving in the bitter Crimea could guard against neuralgia._

ROMANCING THE STUBBLE

Facial hair rules OK in the creative professions and has done ever since Not Shaving became a hallmark of funky chic, as noted by style watcher Peter York back in 1984. Not Shaving has been elevated beyond that negative expression of contrived carelessness affected by superstars such as Dustin Hoffman or Jack Nicholson who can afford to go about looking as if they were just let out of Alcatraz, because everyone knows they're booked into a de luxe Waldorf or a Ritz. Nowadays, as you well know, the Not Shaving syndrome is called Designer Stubble and it's cultivated to give fashionable faces a surface interest that betokens too much intrigue and high-flown business in hand to get into hot water and shaving cream.

Don Johnson of the US television programme _Miami Vice_ is of course a prime suspect. Bob Geldof's Designer Stubble goes hand in hand with his shambled-suit look. When it came to saving the world and our starving children, grooming became an irrelevance, a conceit. So, in time, studied lack of grooming came to acquire a popular romantic appeal, notably among hairdressers, photographers and fashion designers.

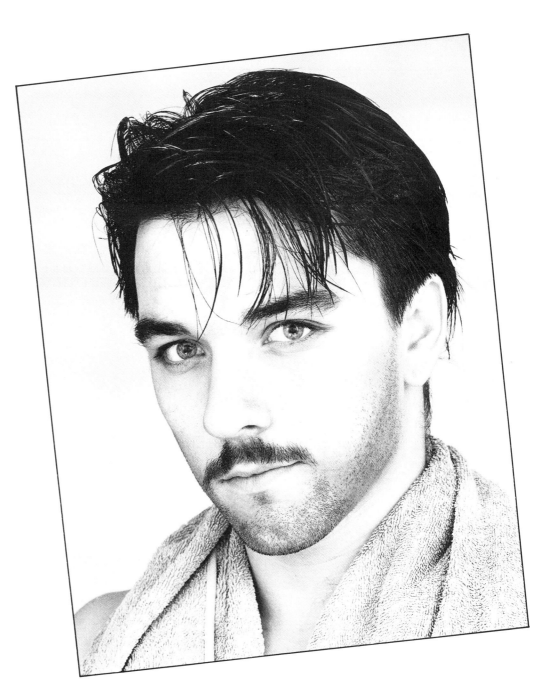

F
A
C
E

SPORTING SPIKES But there still remain sound practical reasons for Not Shaving – even though many of the men who don't shave would run a mile from being dubbed designer material. Rugby players, for instance, particularly props in the front row, prefer to go three or four days without shaving if possible, and they certainly won't go near a razor on the match day itself: even minimal stubble provides some protection against chafing when two faces in the scrum rub too close for comfort.

Martial arts exponents also find stubble a protection against mat burns – an unsightly red rash or positive abrasion that go with taking a tumble. If you study a boxer's face as he weighs in for a match you may well detect a haggard look accentuated by his Not Having Shaved for several days beforehand. Again the resulting growth is thought to provide proof against cuts – as well as a kind of psychological briar barrier! Some boxers – Britain's Barry McGuigan and John Bumphus of the US for two, sport moustaches. Beards also are permitted – just about (Marvin Hagler, US middleweight boxer, has a goatee to complement his bald top) – but only if very well trimmed. Bushy 'Grizzly Adams' styles are definitely not allowed.

IF AT FIRST YOU DON'T SUCCEED Some men simply find it harder than others to develop a luxuriant growth. And some men find it easier to grow a beard at some stages in their lives than others. Changing hormones may play a role; it would certainly be sad, though understandable, if an 18 or 19 year-old were to feel dismayed at his failure to add several years and a good beard to his aspect – the best counsel would be to forget it now – and try again later.

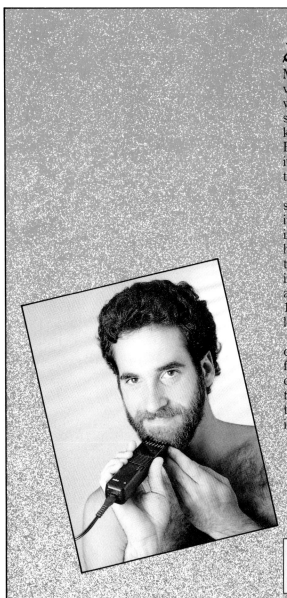

BEAUTY AND THE BEARD

Many members of the bearded fraternity do very nicely, thank you, with a soap and water wash and the occasional trim with whatever scissors happen to be lying around in the kitchen drawer or the household sewing box. Fair enough. But if a thing's worth doing then it's surely worth doing as well as a student of the unsmooth aspect possibly can.

Once your beard's reached the designer stubble stage – and even if you want to keep it at this fairly manicured level, it's worth investing in a beard trimmer. Most electric shavers have a 'long hair' adjustment, but it is possible to buy a beard trimmer with a built-in recharging unit and eight hour charge. It has controls adjustable to four hair lengths: 3mm, 8mm, 14mm and 19mm and can trim a beard of any length claim the manufacturers.

A scissors only man should invest in a decent pair of scissors and keep them strictly for trimming his beard and moustache. Gentle clipping gives far better results than slicing through the undergrowth. If you want to change the length or shape of your beard radically then it's worth going to a professional.

> *A Huguenot admiral liked to use his beard as a pincushion for toothpicks.*

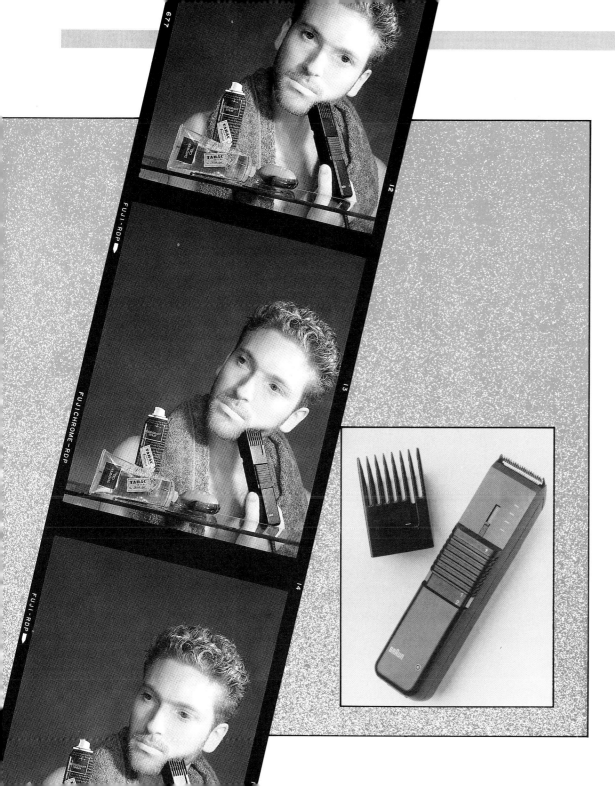

THE COURT CLIPPER The trim treatment can't be better given than by the aptly-named Frank Beard, manager of Truefitt & Hill, who have shaved, trimmed and generally kempt upper-crust men since 1805, when the first Francis Truefitt took premises in London's Old Bond Street (the current salon's at No 23). You can safely take information on the chin from Mr Beard, who in his years as court clipper has trimmed the moustache of actor Sir John Mills and the late Admiral Sir Charles Evans whose gingerish beard "was not quite so tiny as the late conductor Sir Henry Wood's." Not to mention the full set of Prince Michael of Kent, also cared for by Mr Beard who describes it as "a traditional Imperial beard, verging towards the van Dyke with its rounded or almost pointed end. We think it first class."

TRIM AND WEAR IT Mr Beard's style dictum is that the beard on the face is worth two in the mind's eye – in short that it's best to start by looking at the real man and his shape of face, as well as the way his hair grows, rather than beginning with the imagined beard style he thinks he'd like.

"A man's got what he's got", observes Mr Beard plainly. "His hair grows in a certain manner which he'll basically have to accept if he wants a beard at all." It's a question of trim and wear it. You can say you want a pointed goatee, but some men's growth lends itself to this style more than others. It's certainly true that almost all men have a reasonable growth on their chins at least, but some have a particular shape of jaw and growth that lends itself to one style or another. So you can shape but not necessarily style at will.

And shape is the operative word – you don't cut, you gently clip, as you might a fine hedge, hoping – and it's particularly difficult if you're conducting the operation on your own beard or moustache – to keep both sides the same.

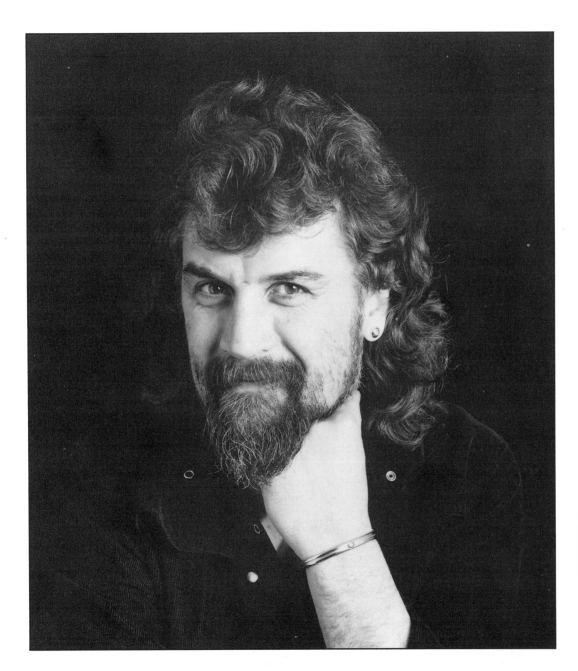

HAIR HORRORS Certain styles Mr Beard cannot abide: "I preferred the more traditional, recognizable styles" he says. "Today there's a lot of fancy-ness which I don't much like". He finds beards that rim the chin with shaven cheeks, trimmed high under the neck, look "too terrible." Cultivated elongated sidepieces down the face look "a little too much of the dandy", any full beard with shaven neck looks "a little bit common" and woe betide the man who lacks the finesse to know that you should never sport beard without moustache.

As far as suiting the growth to face shape is concerned, Frank Beard advocates a fuller beard for fleshing out a thin face, but adds the caveat that if you quite suddenly lose a lot of weight, then a previously well-proportioned beard might make you look "all hair". Also the "new image" impulse prompts you to a complete change: with a new lithe body you hope to discover a complete new you. Shave off the beard, slough off the kilos and start again.

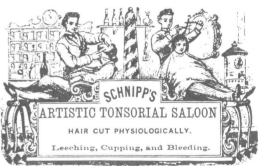

SCHNIPP'S
ARTISTIC TONSORIAL SALOON
HAIR CUT PHYSIOLOGICALLY.
Leeching, Cupping, and Bleeding.

MOUSTACHE MATTERS Frank Beard's own moustache is white with a gentle upturn at each end designed to give his face a slight lift. This lift he says has the effect of lightening one's face and giving you a more cheerful, bonhomous look. Not so the droopy Viva Zapata moustache, which is really a bit sixties-passé and conveys on the wearer a lugubriousness, as if he's Pluto slinking away from the leftovers of a leg of lamb he ought not to have devoured.

DRESSING DOWN AND COLOURING UP Naturally curly and wildly flamboyant moustachioes of the grand old colonel type are now rarely seen outside the theatre. Even the style of bicycle handlebars from which such facial floribunda took their name have changed. Also gone is the preparation known as Bear's Grease (legend does not record what the stuff really contained) which once kept moustaches in control.

Mr Beard has a sneaking suspicion that some gentlemen may even have resorted to dripping as a kind of beard dressing. But all that was in the days before *Pomade Hongroise*, now acknowledged as the best French dressing a beard or moustache can have. Sold either in white (which is really neutral) or blonde, *chataigne* (chestnut), brown or black to tint at your pleasure, the pomade is basically a light grease that keeps your moustache neat and tidy and can assist the upward or downward curl you may favour. Although not permanent, the colour is water-resistant, Mr Beard promises *Pomade Hongroise* doesn't stain or run.

> French chauffeurs formed a Moustache Union in 1911 when their employers pronounced moustaches for servants "presumptuous".

BACK TO THE BARE FACTS – SHAVING IF OFF

As with the beard's initial growth, so with its drastic removal it's worth sounding out your nearest and dearest beforehand. Shocked – even deeply hostile – reactions may follow your change of countenance. Don't be surprised either if some folk fail to notice what you've done, though they may comment vaguely that you look different. It's a measure of just how unobservant we can be!

Frank Beard of Truefitt & Hill (whose salon is pictured below), reckons it takes him about half an hour to take a full beard off. He takes it down first with salon clippers – you could use scissors, but spare the electric shaver the first attack on your hairy layer – it could be more than the finest machine tool can take. Then it's time for a good wet shave. Mr Beard says that contrary to popular claims, the skin buried beneath the bush for who knows how long should not appear shellshocked, pale and greenishly subterranean. It might well have benefitted from a long rest! Shave with particular care for soreness over the first few days. Balms rather than astringent aftershaves are probably best at this stage.

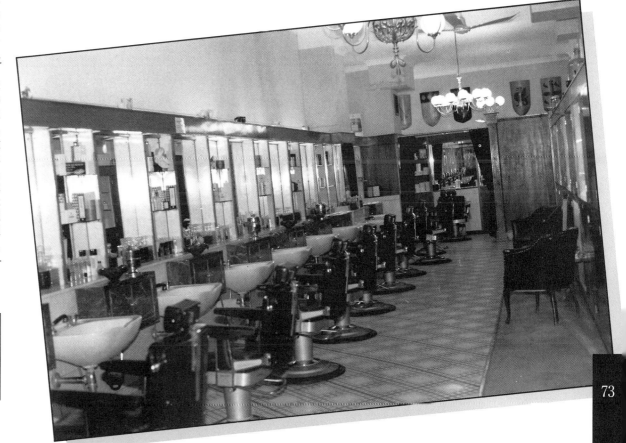

*F*acing *the facts*

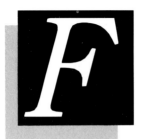

In the beginning, man as a warm-blooded mammal evolved from amphibious ancestors, and he still needed a coat of hair for heat conservation, for camouflage and sun protection. Not until man became a creature of the plains rather than the jungle did his natural hair shirt drop off, leaving his skin side outside. By then he'd developed an effective interior thermostat system – sweat glands connected to the surface by small spiral tubes, a network of surface blood vessels to help him keep cool and extra layers of fat beneath the skin to entrap warmth.

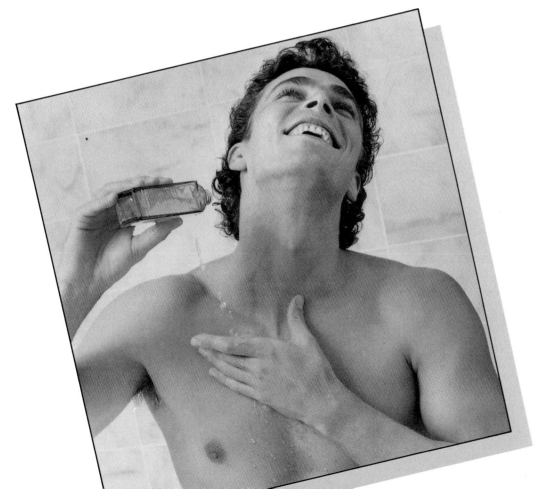

*H*OW DEEP IS SKIN DEEP?

Beauty, as the old maxim says, may only be skin deep, but skin is yours for keeps and is by no means a bland impassive outer casing: like a chameleon its changing colour will reflect emotions surging beneath the skin: anger and embarrassment produce a scarlet face; fright turns one white as the proverbial sheet; pain produces an ashen look and excess expense dinners may leave you a bilious green. Fitness through exercise can also be detected by the shade of your bare-faced cheek: if you exercise strenuously, your temperature rises and the blood vessels in the skin open up so warm blood is close to the cooling outside air. You will then look anything from gently pink to frankly scarlet. In cold weather, the blood vessels contract and divert blood through short circuits to conserve heat. Unless you've been roasting chestnuts over an open fire, this is the time of year you look most pale.

> *The average man has approximately one and a half square metres of skin.*

Looking after the skin is wise because skin is also the real point of human contact, and a focus for sensual attraction. A cross-curled lip may be worth giving the slip but a soft moistened mouth often fires desire. It's a meaningful gesture of affection, of consolation or of just wanting to keep in touch when your beloved puts out a hand to stroke your face – better for her to encounter a soft supple surface than a mock-reptilian casing that might have been dredged from the Great Limpopo River.

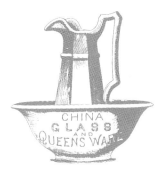

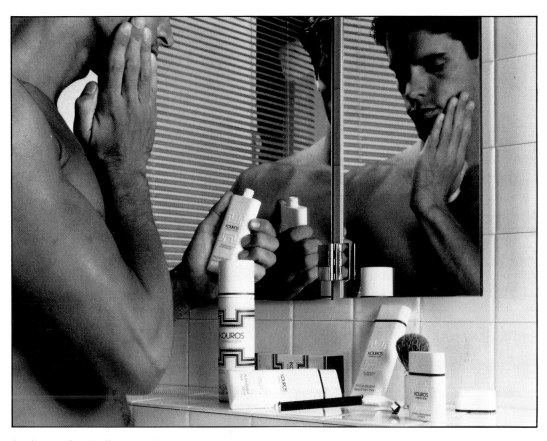

HEALTH BEFORE BEAUTY

But it's not just your looks you protect when caring for your skin. Skin is the body's fine outer armour – a protection against the physical strains of the outside world – wind, weather, air pollution, and the effects of central heating. Your skin is designed also to stop the body beneath drying out, and acts as a defence against the sun's dangerous ultra-violet light. But skin is not entirely impervious – just as sweat is exuded so ointments and creams applied can work their purpose, filtering through the surface skin layer or epidermis to the dermis or lower layers beneath.

Nor is it a fixed organ, in the way you might think of your liver or your lungs. The skin has its own 21–28 day life cycle, which will slow with ageing, but is in effect a constant process of renewal and refreshment. New cells form at the deepest dermal level and are gradually propelled towards the surface where they're shed – quite visibly if your skin is dry and a gentle rub sends flakes flying off into the atmosphere. It's actually claimed that 90 per cent of household dust consists of dead, shed skin.

**F
A
C
E**

MEN'S HEAD START IN THE FACE RACE

Many men only begin to acquire wrinkles ten years after their womenfolk. Some people say that men's skins look better for longer because they're not abused with heavy oil-based creams from an early age as are women's. Men's creams do tend to be lighter and water, rather than oil, based, but there's also a physiological cause for the super-skinned male. If you consider the skin as a well-sprung mattress then its biological springs are collagen and elastin. Men have a thicker outer skin than women and it contains more collagen – perhaps up to 13 per cent more, so that the skin is kept elastic and springy for additional years.

DISHING THE DIRT

But just because nature has been kind with its apportioning of collagen spoils, it doesn't mean you can slap on a bit of soap and forget the rest.

It seems to be a matter of false foolish pride with too many men that each night they give the old teeth a perfunctory one-two with an ancient brush, splash some water in the vague direction of the head, dab with a towel and leap into bed with Len Deighton (in paperback, of course.) All this while the lady of the house is busy with cotton wool and cleansers, with toners and night creams. She is not just wiping off the make-up that took her through the last twelve hours, she is cleaning.

Whilst not wishing any man to turn overnight into a peacock, it is at least worth considering that what is skin sauce for the goose, may also do something for the gander. Cleanliness of the face is not only next to godliness; its good health and good looks sense too, to get rid of surface dirt, to remove the day's detritus and to loosen clogged pores. You don't have to follow a multi-step regime necessarily, but even if you keep your cleaning simple, it's worth being a little scientific and a lot more regular in your approach to upkeep.

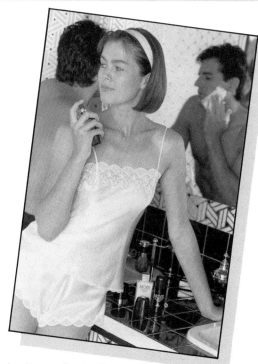

SCRUBBING UP

Another ideal treatment for men's skins, especially those that don't have the benefit of daily skin care, is the exfoliating scrub. It's a granular cleanser which, when removed from the face, should bring with it the dead surface skin cells, oil and dirt, blackheads and other impurities. By stimulating the circulation and cell renewal a good facial scrub should leave your skin with the healthy glow that, in real life, we often have to work quite hard for. Some experts recommend using a face scrub before shaving for a very special occasion, as removal of embedded grime will help the bristles stand well on end. Regular exfoliation also helps to prevent ingrowing hairs on neck and face.

But be warned – exfoliation is not the answer to every man's skin problem – dry skin, sensitive skin, even skin unused to the vigorous onslaught of grains, may become sore and inflamed.

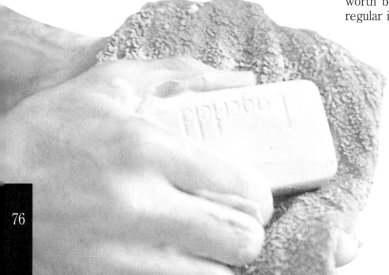

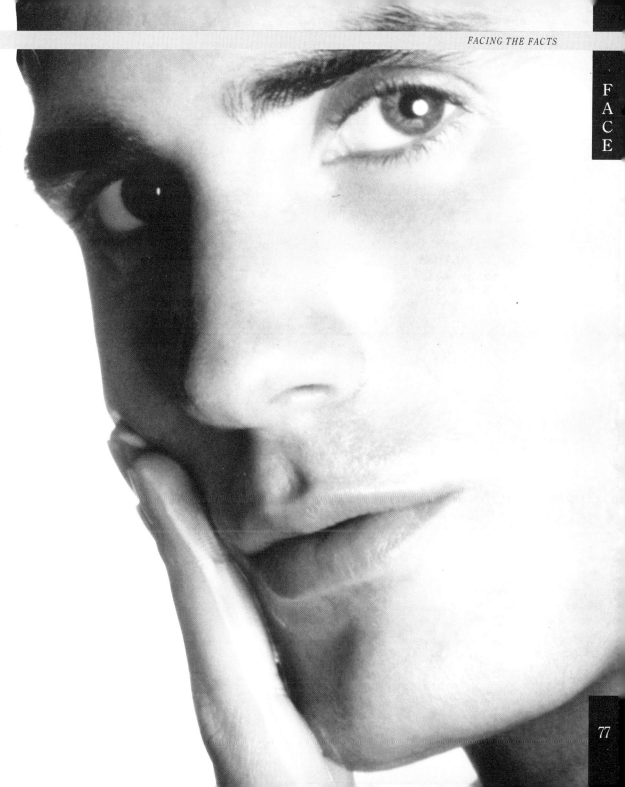

SOFT SOAPING? There's absolutely nothing wrong with the good old basic means of cleansing. If you have strong trouble-free skin you probably can lather in any old soap, but don't even think of doing so if your skin is at all dry or feels tight and sore after a soapy wash. Then you need to abandon ordinary toilet soap and try branded baby soap that's lower in perfume level. There are plenty of specialist soaps for sensitive skins on the market.

For the many oily-skinned men soap-free cleansing bars may be worth a try, and they're also useful for young men whose excessive oiliness is a strong contributory cause of acne. There are specialist soaps on the market which are scientifically prepared for the face. They are recommended for use both night and morning – a regular strength for dry or average skin, extra strength for greasy.

Whatever you use, do try to remember that you are not scrubbing barnacles off a resistant boat hull. Be a little gentle: use warm rather than hotter-than-hell or ice-cold water (which might rupture tiny blood vessels fretworking you with red veins). And remember that if your skin is at all sensitive, fingers may do less irritating harm than flannels.

PORE MAN'S BURDEN – DEEPER CLEANSING Air pollution and central heating alike are enemies of the skin, leaving it dirty and devitalized. So whether you're an indoor or outdoor type, the elements are out to get you. If your skin is greasy then secretions of yellow sebum can clog up the pores on the skin surface (especially common on men's noses) which then look particularly large and unappealing. Any bacteria trapped in these pores turn them black – and blackheads are decidedly not beautiful.

To prevent the dull dry look, or the blackhead-bridged nose it's no bad idea to give your face a more thorough cleanse daily with a facewash or cleansing milk.

F
A
C
E

PROFESSIONAL SPRING CLEAN

Time was when macho man took off the greasy shine with the fiercest of exfoliators – pumice, or even a loofah. Now the smart solution is to go to a professional skincare expert for a facial. Beauty therapists observe that even though men are initially more reluctant to lie back on the couch and submit to massaging ministrations, they tend to be more appreciative of the relaxation and end improvement a good facial puts their way. If you're looking for a facial, the rule seems to be that hair salons which cater for both sexes and also have beauty treatment rooms make no sexual discrimination.

MOISTURE MECHANICS

Water may not be the most exciting liquid you can name, but it's the ingredient essential for a smooth, pliant skin. If you're happy enough with the texture of a dessicated coconut, read no further. But the fact is that good-looking, youthful skin holds up to an astonishing fourteen pints of water. About 8 per cent of this lies in the epidermis, which presents its face to the outside world, and which helpful skin care products can penetrate. But roughly 3 and a half pints of water is lost through the skin each day. Air conditioning and office block central heating do nothing to minimize this loss, so it's up to you to help put back what the environment takes out.

Toiletry manufacturers have racked their brains for a less effeminate name than 'moisturizer' to give the ever-increasing variety of creams they commend to your daily use. Some have added the tag 'aftershave' in the hope that if you apply the cream as part of your razor routine you won't feel you're betraying your masculinity. But moisturizing creams are really what they're offering – and what you need.

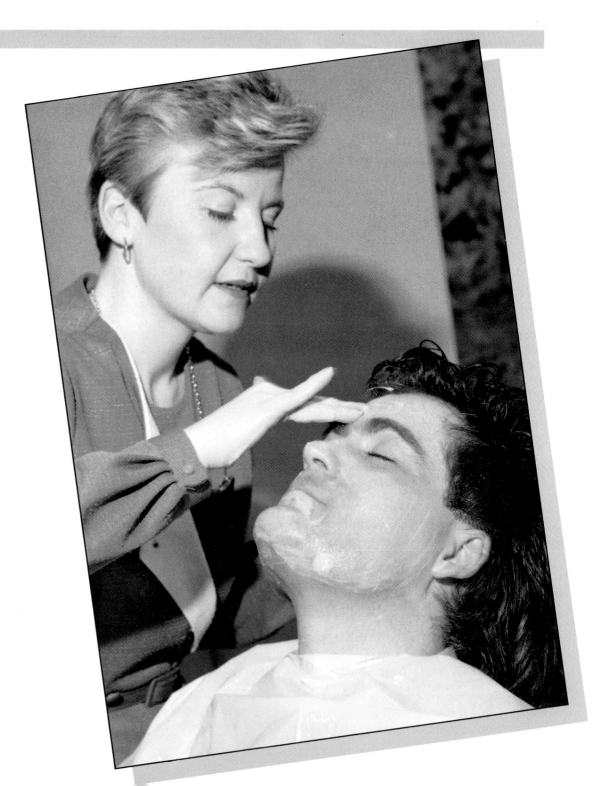

At Leonard's in London's Mayfair, you can have a 50 minute facial and massage for less than the price of two good theatre tickets. Trained therapists cleanse, tone and exfoliate, using Clarins products before exposing your world-weary face to an ozone steamer, opening the pores so that blackheads, whiteheads and tiny fatty cells or 'millia' under the skin surface can be easily removed with deep cleanse or, if necessary, a very fine needle (no, they promise it won't hurt.) Then there's toning and application of revitalizing aromatherapy oils. A 20 minute facial massage improves the circulation and lymphatic drainage. Then it's on with a face mask, more cleanse and tone and a light oil finish before you're on your way, having lost your tension along with the dead skin.

Judging by the tell-tale tubes tucked away in sports bags and briefcases it does seem to be catching on. And the moisturizer-makers do seem to have cottoned on to the fact that men want a light, easily-absorbed, invisible all-purpose cream for easy use after a squash match and ensuing shower, after a hasty battery shave before an evening date, or coming in from a run in the skin-battering wind and rain. They ought, of course, to put it on before braving the wind and the rain as extra protection.

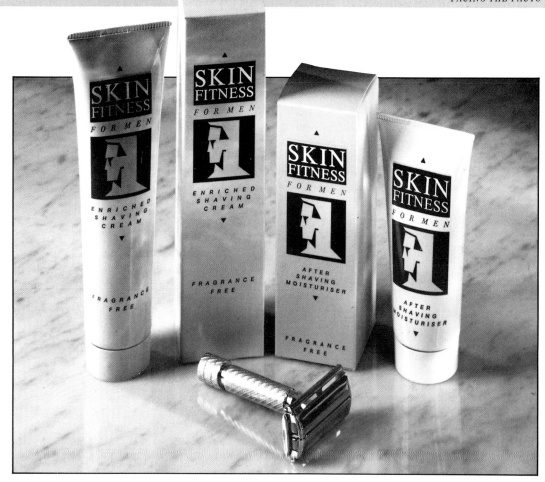

YOUTH DUE Some moisturizers contain a substance called collagen which is claimed to have rejuvenating properties, but there seems to be an ongoing division between doctors and dermatologists who pour scorn on long term rejuvenating benefits of collagen applied to the skin and the skincare producers who heartily commend it. But certainly those who've tried a good moisturizing cream or aftershave balm claim instant relief from dryness, and soreness, and within a day or two find their skins feel generally more supple. And that, in the end, is what counts more than any attempt to blind you with impressive scientific lowdown. One

American professor of dermatology, Professor Albert Kligman, who is regarded as a guru of skin care, crusades for the daily use of nothing more exotic than good old household petroleum jelly.

FEEDING YOUR FACE

Dietary doyens offer the constant reminder that "you are what you eat". By now everyone knows that you are best-fed on plenty of fresh green vegetables and fruit, raw salads, limited red meat, no added salt and a sufficiency of fibre, not to mention your fair share of vitamins.

FACE

The vitamins your face needs

VITAMIN A (plentiful in dairy products, carrots and tomatoes), guards against dry, rough skin and irrigates the eyes.

VITAMIN B2 (present in liver, milk and green vegetables), prevents dry, cracked lips and sores in the corner of the mouth.

The Vitamin B group contains nicotinic acid (meat, fish, pulses and wholemeal provide it), stops your skin becoming sensitive to sunlight, stops it darkening in colour too, and forming unsightly scales.

VITAMIN C (found in fresh fruit and vegetables), aids healing of wounds and keeps gums healthy.

VITAMIN D (found in fish liver oils, milk and eggs), keeps bones healthy and is actually made by the skin from sunlight.

VITAMIN E (usually taken as capsule supplement available from health food stores), is the most controversial of the bunch. At least one US dermatologist, Dr Samuel Ayres, is recommending its intake as acne treatment. Vitamin E is also said to be an anti-ageing agent. Those who use it swear by it, those who don't think it quackery.

Don't be defective in other dietary essentials:

Calcium: (cheese, milk, oranges, nuts and carrots) helps guard against dry skin.

Iron: (present in spinach, watercress, cabbage, carrots and cereals) is the Popeye supplement that keeps your blood in good, oxygenated order. Too little iron can cause anaemia.

If you're healthy and taking anything other than an extremely poor diet of endless chips and cups of tea, you should not need any additional vitamin supplements. If in doubt, don't spend and swallow, consult your doctor.

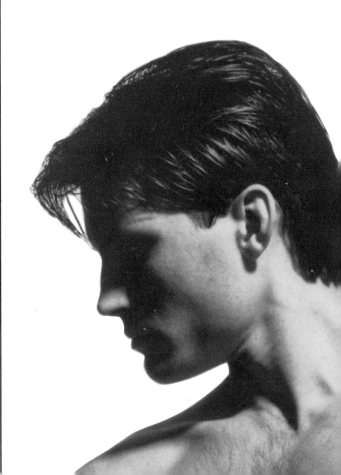

F
A
C
E

FAST FOOD The real problem about being what you eat, is that you are also what you do. Which is probably too much too fast to leave a great deal of time for eating, let alone preparing salads of raw cabbage, walnuts and cottage cheese. Fast food may be to your taste as well as your convenience, but try to counteract the effect of endless burgers and fried chicken pieces with some raw fruit or vegetables each day. The bad news about fast, or any other processed (tinned, packaged, preserved) foods is that they sometimes clog up the system and cause constipation. And when the gut fails to eliminate unwelcome waste products, that's when your skin is prone to break out, and generally give itself a dull, apathetic look. Perhaps the best dietary advice is to notice what food makes you feel – and look – good, and what discomforts and upsets you. It's a question of using sense tempered by appetite.

A CHOC BAR A DAY? Dermatologists are now saying that most skin problems have nothing to do with diet. Research tests on both sides of the Atlantic have failed to find any real correlation between the chocaholic and his acne. You might improve a spotty skin if you adopted an extremely low-fat diet over a long period but this should only be after specialist advice. Cutting down on dairy foods might help some people, but if you develop a crop of spots following a raid on the sweet shop, guilt-induced stress rather than sugar may be the cause. Sugar will probably do more harm to your teeth than to your skin.

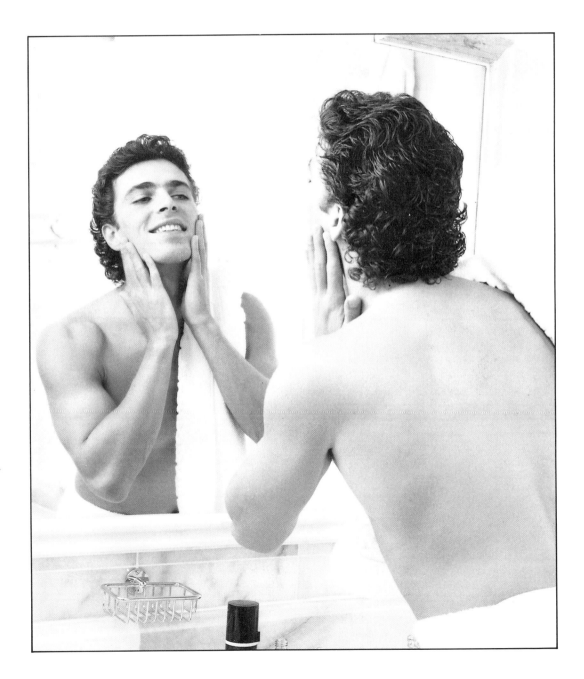

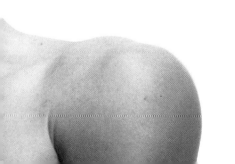

BOOZE IS BAD FOR YOU An ancient Roman inscription above the Pump Room, Bath, reads "Water is best". Too true, tap or mineral, sparkling or flat, drinking plenty of water is super for the skin – a pore man's champagne. Alcohol, however, is fattening, yet offers absolutely nothing in the way of vitamin or mineral nutrients. It could stimulate your appetite so you want to eat more. It positively strips you of Vitamin B and can leave you with bloodshot eyes the next morning, not to mention a tracery of fine red veins in years to come. Beware the facial fate of Sebastian Flyte, of Evelyn Waugh's *Brideshead Revisited*, in whom alcohol 'wrought the change of years. . . He was paler, thinner, pouchy under the eyes, drooping in the corners of his mouth, and he showed the scars of a boil on the side of his chin.' There's no need to be teetotal – just be temperate, and remember that the better a wine, the less harm it's likely to do you: it's the house plonk that decants most toxic substances into your cells.

Smoking may not only damage your general health but inhibit your power to absorb vitamin C, and impair good skin circulation by contracting the blood vessels. Shortage of vitamin C could damage your collagen – which is why so many smokers reach wrinkles sooner than their nicotine-free friends.

SKIN ALIVE Your best present to your face is your best present to the rest of you too. It's a balanced – and that doesn't mean boring – lifestyle, incorporating exercise, good meal sense, adequate sleep and plenty of good times to make you glow.

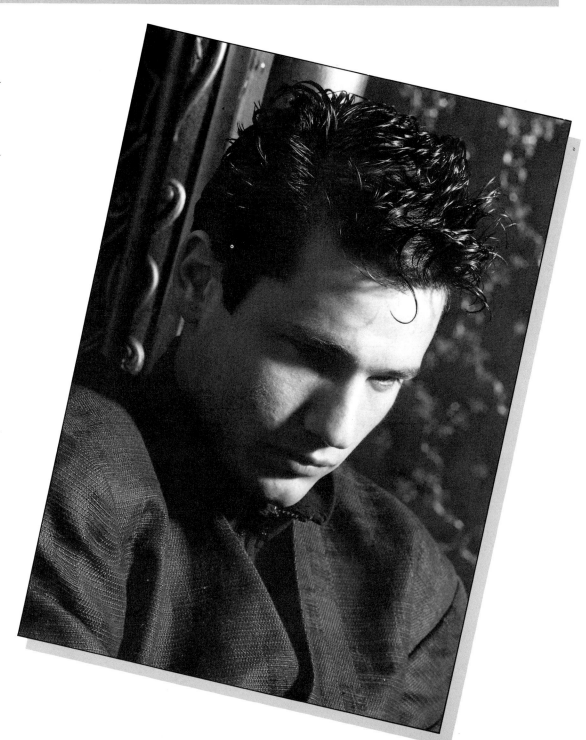

BREAKING OUT – THE FACE THAT LAUNCHED A THOUSAND ZITS

Acne is awful, but you are not alone with the problem: about half the teenage population develops some form of acne, which accounts for around 15 per cent of all doctors' consultations each year. Most acne sufferers will grow out of their spots and reach adulthood unscarred, but in one unfortunate man in every 100 between the age of 25 and 40, the condition persists.

Basically your acne is caused by a rush of hormonal action, most often triggered by adolescence. Over-production of sebum – a fatty secretion – can clog up the sebaceous glands, which may become inflamed and at worst, infected. The actual spots are caused by bacteria collecting beneath the clogged area.

Although keeping the surface skin clean does nothing to confront the underlying cause, it will keep down the top layer of grease that collects and could cause blackheads. Wash twice daily with a clear glycerine (rather than fatty) soap. Use tissues to wipe off, rather than a flannel which could re-infect on re-use. Don't, whatever you do, pick and worry at the spots, which will spread the infection or cause scarring – the permanent acne blemishes you want at all cost to avoid.

It's very difficult to recommend a single course of action against acne as it's a highly individual complaint, with no single cure. At least now the dermatologists are on your side and the psychological pain of pimples is understood. What outsiders may view as three or four spots, you, the victim, may blow up in your imagination to a plague of pustules. The rule of thumb should be that if you feel bad about them – act. Don't be put off by kindly veterans ascribing it to your age, and if your doctor fails to give you the help you need, ask to see a specialist. Equally, avoid over-reaction: there are still non-medical, private clinics who will peel your skin with drastic abrasive chemicals. Have none of this.

A do-it-yourself peeling with a sulphur and resorcinol paste from the chemist is, however, worth a try, as is a benzoyl peroxide cream. Your first line of defence should be to understand the problem – and to keep a curb on the misery it induces: stress could aggravate it. Don't fight what you can't change, just take sensible measures to keep your face clean and seek expert help.

Seeking early help for severe acne also minimizes the risk of permanent skin damage. But don't expect results overnight, because any reputable skin specialist will want to try the gentlest remedy before working his way up to more drastic treatment. Even a straightforward course of tetracyclin antibiotics takes time to work, possibly as long as six months.

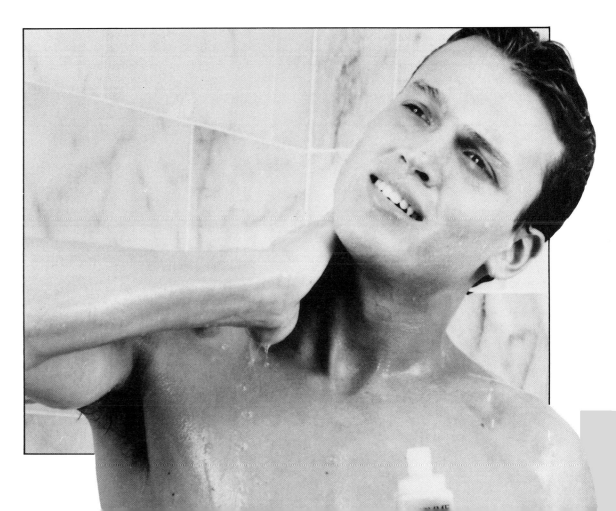

OUT, OUT DAMN SPOT

BLACKHEADS Are caused by dirt and grime lodging in a clogged pore and can be kept down by attentive cleaning. But having a go at those already present calls for clean steady hands. Warm your face with a very clean, hot flannel or by leaning over a basin full of very hot water to soften the skin, then squeeze the blackheads with care, using clean fingertips and tissues. Don't pinch it from the top, but work away downwards and beneath. At worst you may need to stretch the skin area slightly to bring the blackhead out. If you're hopelessly inept, don't persevere with this technique; ask a loved one or take yourself for a professional facial.

WHITEHEADS Are another form of tiny obstructing skin plugs, most visible when the skin around them is stretched. They're not as amenable as blackheads to home treatment and can lead to acne spots. Cleaning regularly to keep the oily surface to a minimum is the best defence against their build up.

IMPROVING ON NATURE – THE GREAT ILLUSIONS

If grades were given for grooming effort, most women would probably score A minus; most men, at least until recently, C plus. Men's disinclination to improve upon nature can't however be put down to laziness alone, nor yet indifference. It's much more likely to be a matter of Negative Image Management. The average man will not care to be seen – warts and all – any more than a woman would. But times are changing and there is an increasing readiness, amongst men, to enhance existing assets and use a little illusion on facial deficits.

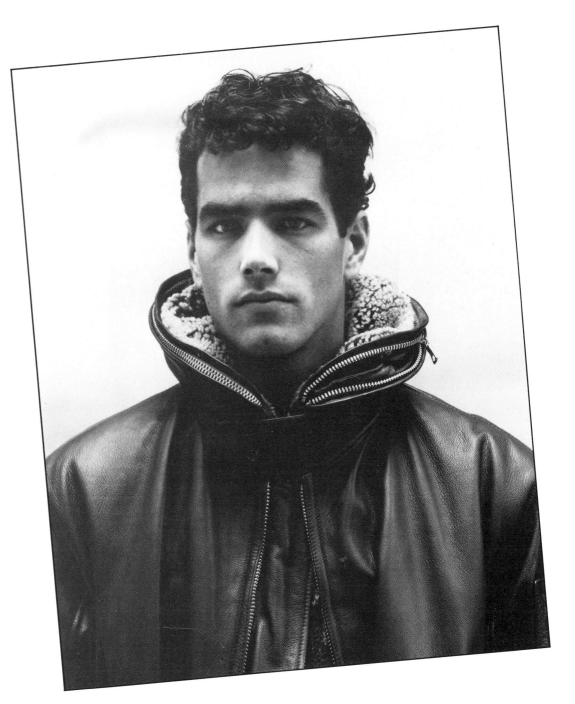

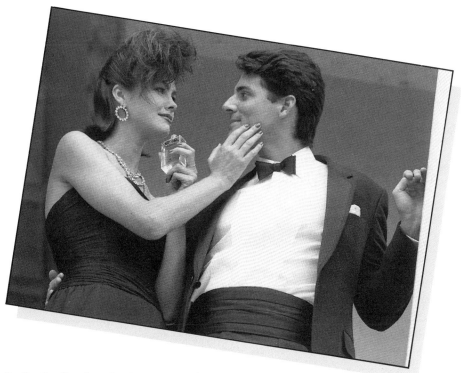

JOIN THE BROWNIES

"Bronzers", snorted a man so conservative he wouldn't be smelt with a dab of cologne behind his ears, "They're strictly for the very callow young, for woofters and sick executives who believe that brown is good for business." Such prejudice should have gone out with the slave trade. Nobody's suggesting you stripe up like David Bowie or blacken your lips like Boy George, but a touch of tan can certainly give a fillip to a washed-out February face and lift you out of the pale doldrums at the dog-end of the year.

It's no longer news that too much sybaritic lying about in the sun harms the skin both short and long-term. Yet paradoxically a suntan is still a certain status symbol. Using a bronzer is an obvious way of resolving this contradiction with-out paying the health price.

FALSE COLOURS Today's bronzers give instant, short-term special effects. They're usually in gel form, often incorporated into aftershaves and designed to be non-streaky, and completely waterproof for a day's duration. Then you sim-ply wash off with soap and water. The application secret is to squeeze a little on to a wet palm, rub the hands together and spread quickly over the face for all-over cover. Bronzers come in all sorts of guises from the non-streak vari-ety, tinted sports gels, tinted aftershave mois-turizers to moisturizing tanning gels.

With all these products it's best to try them out before an important occasion. Bronzer col-ours can be modified by your own skin tones and it can be quite a shock when what appeared to be golden tan in the tube tarnishes into muddy terra cotta on your face.

HAIRY TALES

Unwanted hair is one of those phrases that strikes dread in the heart of anyone who wants to feel groomed. For men it's far less of a fear than for women, but unexpected and unwel-come sprouting from ears and nose can be vis-ited upon you, especially after the late thirties.

GROW BROW Eyebrows that threaten not just to bush but positively to thicket require some sort of gardening. Eyebrows that meet in the middle (usually dark ones) look positively threatening. Some men seem to relish brows of great character, but if you prefer to be remembered by more graceful features you have the choice of trimming, tweezer-plucking (fine but can be a sore job), or electrolysis.

The process of electrolysis is slow and meticulous. Hairs are removed by the introduc-tion of an electrode or very fine needle into the hair follicle. Immediately after this a short wave current is applied of a fraction of a second to coagulate the papilla at the base of the hair follicle so that the loosened hair can be lifted out. The first stage of this procedure should be painless, and the discomfort of the second stage varies from reported pain, to claims of slight tingling.

Clients are usually treated for a 20 minute period at a time, which allows for some 75–100 hairs to be removed. Although such hair removal is permanent you may experience some regrowth if you've done so much past tweezing (or waxing) that hair follicles have become distorted, and depending on how much current your skin type can withstand. But with each treatment regrowth will weaken and finally cease.

Check that your operator is professionally qualified and approved by The Institute of Elec-trolysis. And make absolutely certain that, with the danger of AIDS and Hepatitis B, fresh nee-dles are used for each treatment.

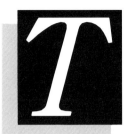eeth and smiles

The hole truth is that you can no longer look to your dentist to do all the work for you. The first responsibility for maintaining your teeth in mint condition lies with you. Preventive Dentistry is the name of the game. Every decent dental practice now has its resident hygienist. Ask for an appointment and have the whys and wherefores demonstrated clearly to you, as follows.

Disclosing tablets or liquid indicate whether you're making a good job of brushing: coloured stains stand out on areas you're missing and where plaque is collecting.

Brush after each meal with small, circular motions right down onto the gums. Take time over the job; using a smaller bristle brush than you're used to often enables you to reach awkward corners at the back of the mouth.

If your teeth and gums are sensitive you should be visiting the hygienist for periodontal treatment every three to six months and possibly using a special preparation toothpaste. Avoid strong tooth powders.

The Government's AIDS advice booklet warns against sharing a toothbrush even with a member of the same family.

Good dental health means that you can cast to the four winds your bottles of breath-sweetening mouthwashes and sprays. These fresheners are only designed to camouflage an underlying problem, and if you've looked after your mouth you won't have the parrot's cage problem that stems from unhealthy gums and neglected teeth.

Dental Floss is the white, waxed string you wrap around two middle fingers and seesaw back and forth between every two teeth in your head, using a different section as you move along the mouth. Flossing effects the final 40 per cent of the teeth cleaning job. Do it daily.

OTHER TOOTH TOOLS Treated tooth picks available from your local chemist's counter massage and so heal sore gums as well as ensuring that resistant food is removed from crevices in your teeth.

Special interspace brushes with tiny bristle heads, like a mini-shaving brush, are very useful for removing plaque from corners of the teeth an ordinary toothbrush cannot reach.

HOLE CONTROL DIET To cut out the sugar is to cut down, if not out, the cavities. Sugar, whether in the form of sweets, sweet or fizzy drinks or fresh fruit juice is out. As soon as sugar makes contact with your teeth it produces acids that rot the enamel. If you must eat sugary foods eat them in one fell swoop; then clean your teeth.

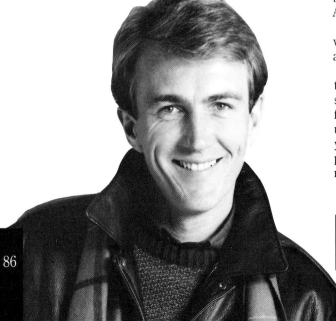

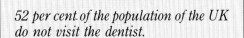

52 per cent of the population of the UK do not visit the dentist.

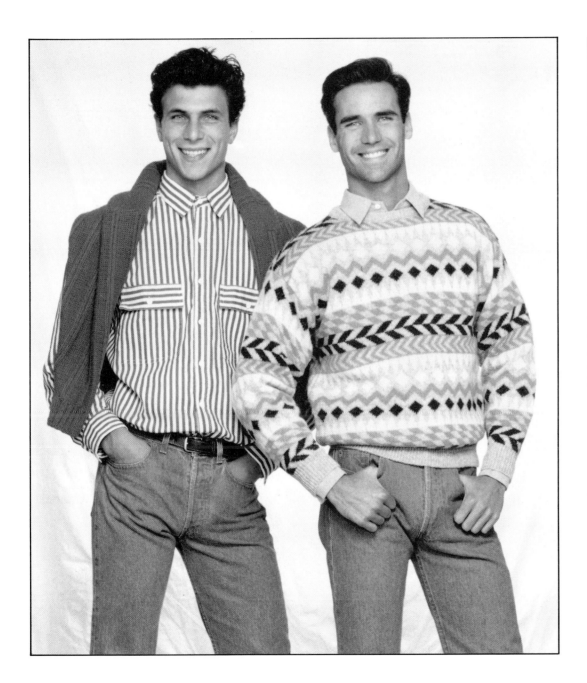

Early 19th century dentures were known as 'Waterloo' teeth; because they were often fashioned from gnashers plundered from graves or battlefields.

1.3 toothbrushes a year is the average rate of exchange. It should be four.

90 per cent of the population suffers from some degree of gum disease.

Taking the Chair

The purpose of your twice-yearly dental check-up is to ensure that no new cavities have appeared. You will also have your teeth descaled and polished so that you come out looking like a grand piano straight out of the showroom window. It's likely to be a minimal affair if you do need a filling – dentists drill the smallest possible areas and fill with tooth-coloured composites designed for hard wear.

It's important to have a dentist you feel free to ask questions. If yours is not amenable to friendly professional discussion or if he makes you feel you've got the most evil set of chompers since Jaws, then change your dentist.

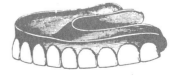

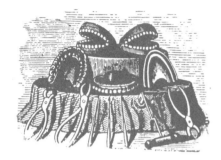

9.3 million people fear the dentist.

More toothpaste is being squeezed: 22,600 tons in 1984, compared with 20,700 in 1980.

In one recent year 33 million teeth were filled, six million teeth extracted, two million were crowned and one and a half million dentures were fitted.

Say "cheese". Cheddar chewed at the end of a meal helps protect the teeth by neutralizing the effect of the foregoing courses.

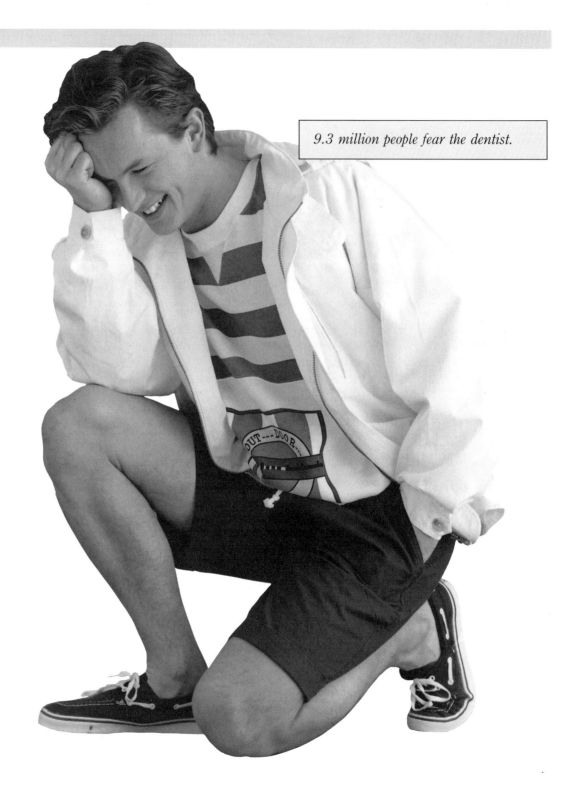

ENGINEERING WORKS

CROWNS OR CAPS Are used to cover up damaged teeth. A broken tooth may be drilled down into a pet shape and covered with a 'jacket crown' blended to match the other teeth. A dead, root-filled tooth can be saved by a 'post crown' with an artificial peg holding it firm to the root.

BRIDGE OVER TROUBLED WATER A gap left by a missing or extracted tooth can be 'invisibly mended' with a bonded porcelain tooth attached by using the adjacent teeth as supporting pillars. Very often they too must be crowned to strengthen them. A new development is the bonded bridge, whereby the adjacent teeth are not crowned but treated with a very mild acid so that their back surface can take metal tags which hold the replacement tooth in place without the need for crowns.

DENTURES Don't ask. The whole purpose of modern dental health care is to render them redundant!

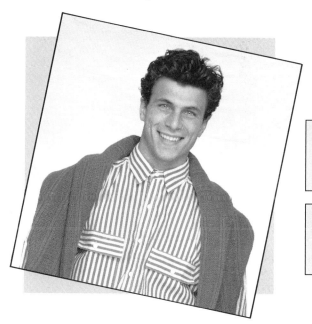

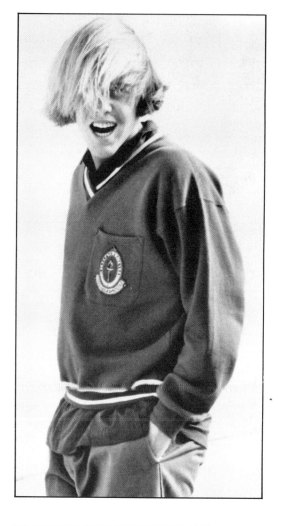

George Washington soaked his false teeth overnight in port. He must have craved a sweet awakening.

The first dentist's drill was patented in 1872, the Morrison treadle-driven dental engine.

Men are less diligent than women about going to the dentist. But by good fortune they keep their teeth several years longer – until the age of 57.

Tea drinkers are less prone to tooth decay than the rest of the population: it's the tannin that does the trick almost as effectively as fluoride. Unless you add sugar, of course. . .

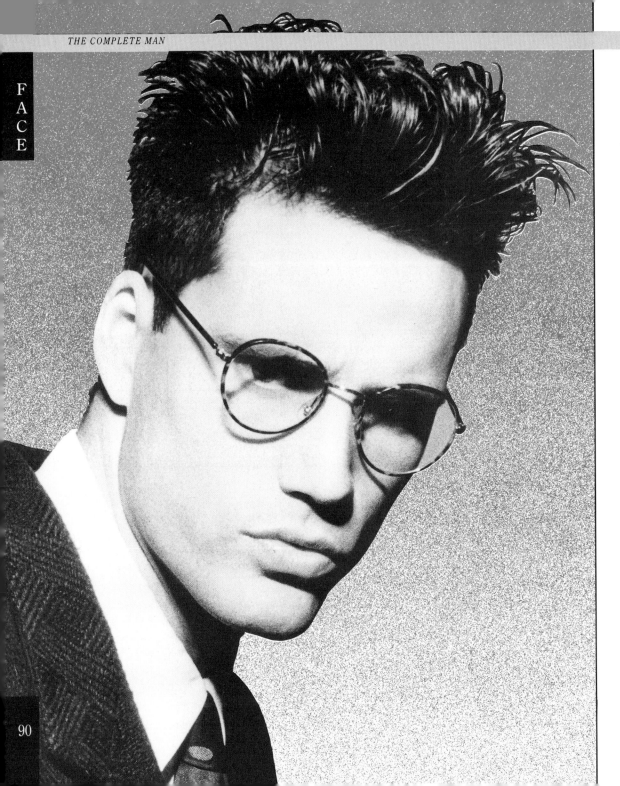

A SIGHT FOR SORE EYES

Smoke gets in your eyes: dust, poor light, too many hours at the VDU screen; city streets, one drink too many; a poor quality film print – any number of environmental and occupational factors can conspire to irritate your oculars. If the whites of your eyes read like a road map what you need is a vasoconstrictor (no relation to the serpentine boa) to shrink the blood vessels back to normal size. The best approach is to prepare a cool compress – cold camomile tea on cotton wool pads works marvels, but if you're in a hurry lay on two cold tea bags and lie down for 10–15 minutes. Chilled cucumber slices or even cotton wool balls dipped in iced water have been recommended by opthalmologists. Compresses are more effective than eye drops.

IN THE LAND OF DARK SHADOWS

Lack of sleep, vitamin deficiencies, or inherited predisposition can ring your eyes with black shadows. If you think you've been abusing your body, have some early nights, take more fresh air and be kind to your overworked system. If you're stuck, like an old-fashioned doctor, with your little black bags, the only option is a concealer stick, a skin coloured cover-up applied with restraint to the darkest rings and blended in well.

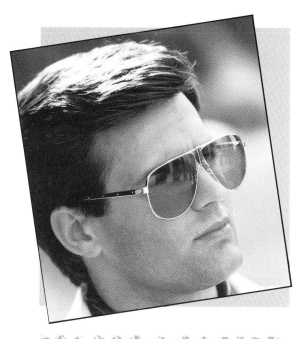

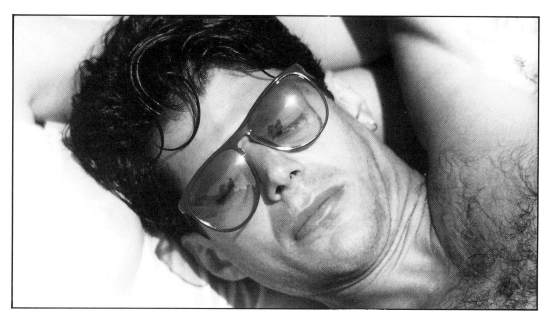

A HINT OF TINT

More men now use hair colour – which leaves their eyebrows and eyelashes looking oddly mismatched, as if on loan from some other gentleman entirely. Fair men sometimes feel that their brows and lashes have faded away altogether and would prefer a stronger outline. The answer in both cases must be a hint of tint on brows and lashes. Don't try doing the job yourself as the eye area is sensitive and the job delicate. Find a professional beauty salon or unisex hairdresser that offers this service. The job takes 20–25 minutes. Special eye tints are used, from a colour choice of black, brown or blue-black. First the hair is peroxided with a very mild solution, which won't hurt, but might make your eyes sting. Then the colour is put on with a small brush or orange stick. You'll remain dark and interesting for four–five weeks.

ON SPEC

The optical trade has come a very long way since the Emperor Nero was left to rely on an emerald ring to magnify his vision. Since glasses are a positive statement, there to be seen as well as to help you see, it's worth choosing with care. Leave the science side to a registered optician and put all your energies and sense of style into choosing frames that complement your face. And don't ever accept it as an inevitable accompaniment to imperfect vision that your nose should be rubbed red and raw on either side. If your glasses pinch, then they don't fit well. Take them back. If you need very heavy lenses for sight correction, this no longer means that you'll require such weighty supporting frames that you end up with a headache. You can try perspex lenses (they scratch but can be reground), and you can also now buy very strong but light plastic frames.

GETTING FRAMED – EYEING UP THE ALTERNATIVES

Rounded frames have a neutral effect on the face, accentuating neither horizontal nor vertical lines.

A horizontal upper rim breaks up vertical lines of a face, and broadens it. This style looks best on long slim faces – and the effect can be heightened if the lower rim is also horizontal.

Downswept outer frames accentuate breadth in the lower half of the face, and give a restful look.

Big wide frames make a face look smaller and can make the nose look thinner too.

Nose shapes can also be modified by the shape of the spectacle bridge: the saddle bridge (particularly comfortable as the frame itself sits on the nose) has a shortening effect on a long conk, a keyhole or padded bridge can appear to lengthen a nose. If you're a bit of a Pinocchio, but want a padded bridge, choose a bridge set further forward and deeper.

Your choice of sidepieces can actually change the look of your profile: thin sidepieces on a heavier plastic frame seem to 'stretch the profile'. Heavier plastic sidepieces reduce the profile and work well on men whose ears are set well back on the head.

THE COLOUR CODE

Traditionally men have fallen for the heavy brown-bottle or imitation tortoiseshell glasses framing. But recent years have seen a real breakthrough in style with a good deal more variety. Matt black is popular, also blues and greys, and men who previously drew the line at any glimmer of glitter, are now much braver about gold trim on face and side pieces. Metal – as opposed to plastic – is lighter in frame construction, but can lend a 'cool' effect, especially in silver chrome, steel or titanium.

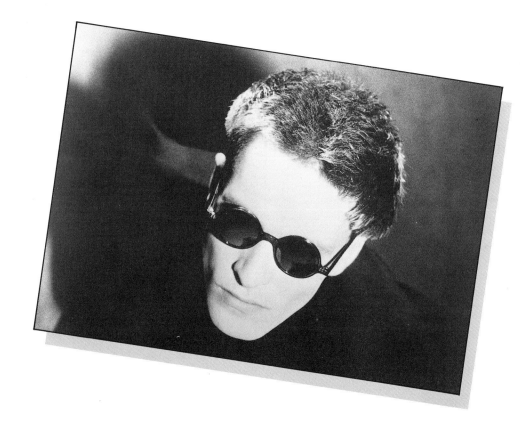

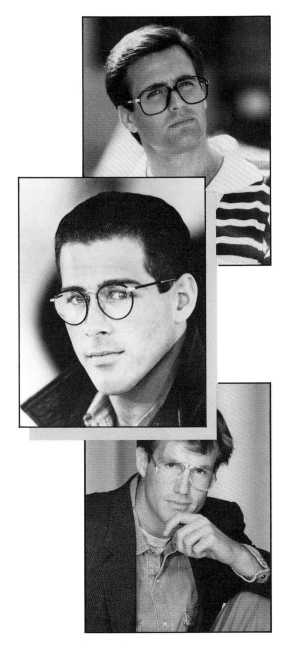

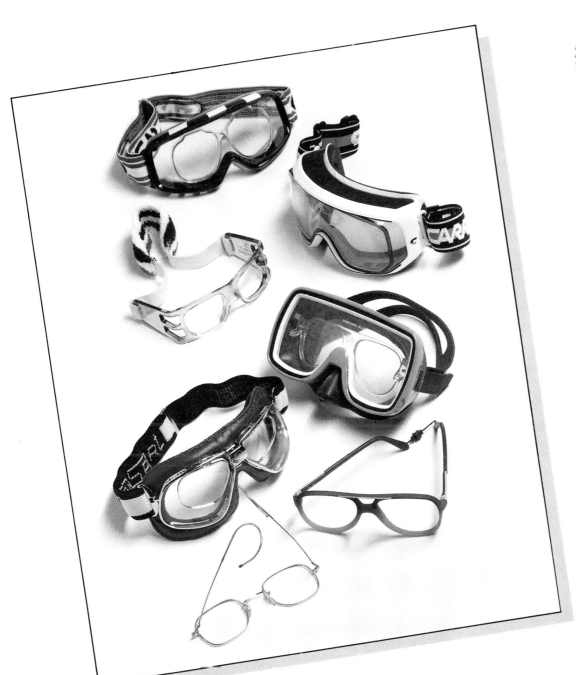

A SPORTS SPECTACLE

If you're an active sportsman you really need a pair of hardwearing sports specs to withstand the extra stresses of varied exercise and to allow an unimpeded, wide field of vision. Look for frames with high set sides, often made from springily pliant metal or tough plastic with sprung hinges.

It's no knockout losing your goggles mid-field, so consider frames with curled metal sides which keep a firmer hold than the ordinary 'hockey stick' ear pieces. You can now buy adjustable sports headbands to attach to your everyday frames, or select a frame purpose-built with integral band. At the very least you should ensure that your eyes are safeguarded by lenses of toughened glass or break-resistant plastic. Polycarbonate lenses made up to pre-scription are more protective for the potentially dangerous tumbles you may take, for instance, whilst out riding.

If you're a squash player you must opt for a wrap-around goggles with face-hugging rub-ber cushioned frame and secure adjustable headband. Have the lenses made up to your prescription.

Scuba specs are also available: you can buy a diving mask with a special frontpiece into which your own prescription lenses can be clip-ped and unclipped.

F
A
C
E

MAKING CONTACT

Contact lenses are tiny, shell-like discs fitted to the front curve of the eye. If you take to them well they're barely detectable, even to an optician, who'd have to peer very closely to find you out.

> *Leonardo da Vinci first sketched the idea of a contact lens as an optical aid back in 1508 – but it took 440 years for the theory to be translated into practice.*

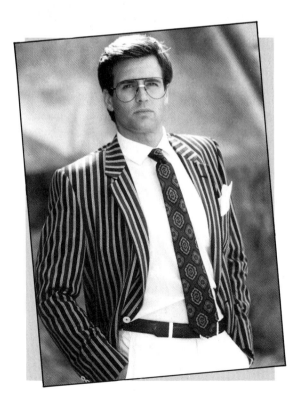

SUIT-EYE-BALL? It's wise to recognize from the first that not everyone is a suitable contact candidate. Good opticians will take a very detailed history from you, to ensure that your eyes are not too sensitive, are well-lubricated and that your particular lens prescription can be translated into contacts.

LENS LORE Traditional hard contact lenses are the budget buy, but they limit oxygen supply to the eye and can irritate the wearer in smoke or bright-lit conditions. They can't be worn for very many hours at a time.

Gas permeable lenses let oxygen through, feel more comfortable and can therefore be worn for longer at one stretch. At present they're often the lens of first choice.

Soft lenses offer great comfort, and are much easier to adjust to. But they're far more fragile, inclined to tear and unlikely to last much beyond eighteen months to two years.

Hard lens wearers will be advised to put them in for no more than two hours a day, working up by the hour over a few weeks. Soft lens wearers will adapt much faster – they can usually wear their lenses for four to six hours a day straight off increasing to eight to ten hours after a few days.

Don't forget to sterilize your lenses daily with the recommended preparation – a leading optician thought it rather served the gent. right who went to lick his lens clean, but swallowed by mistake! Saliva contains bacteria – your eyes should not! It's also unwise to depend solely on one pair of contact lenses to see you through. You'll need a back up pair of glasses – if only to grope fruitfully about on the floor in search of the lens you accidentally dropped. . .

FACE SHAPE SENSE

A Square Face can either be played up by the addition of equally strong square frames. Alternatively play down the jaw line with slightly curved or rounded glasses and a little height on the top rim.

A Long Face needs frames to add width; round sides and horizontal lower rims add contour.

A Round Face could do with a touch of the geometrics – frames cut straight across the top, angling in towards the lower rim and squared off again. Choose frames that tilt up slightly to accentuate the cheekbones and focus attention away from global jowls.

A Triangular Face with broad forehead and tapering chin is best set off by thin frames and dominant vertical lines.

An Oval Face is the ideal shape to be blessed with. Take your choice from the optician's gallery.

But don't, whatever your face shape, job or lifestyle be swayed overmuch by fashion. Suit yourself, not external trends.

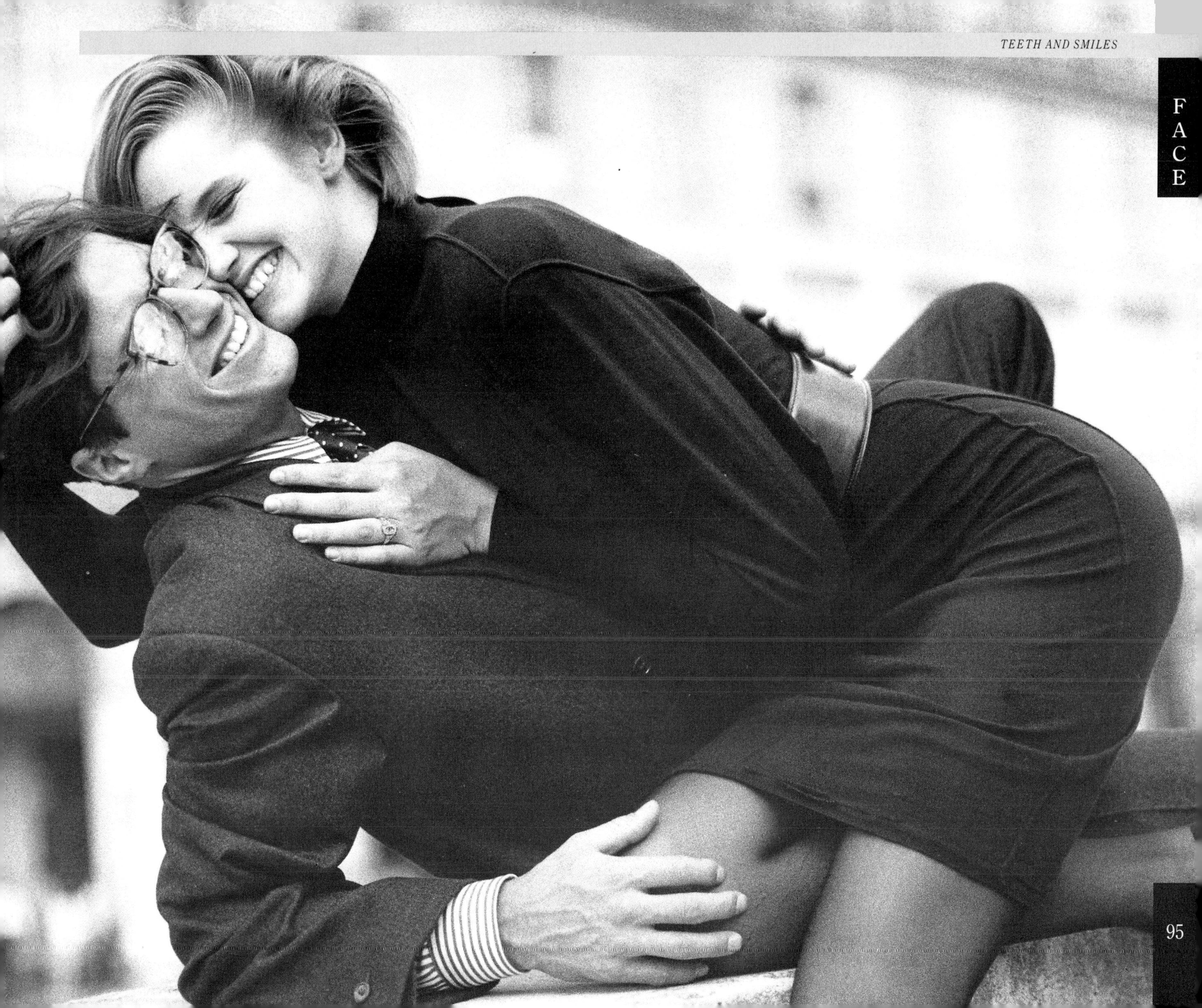

Weather or not

SKIN VERSUS THE ELEMENTS

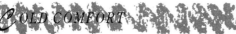

COLD COMFORT

It's easy to feel trapped by a seasonal vicious circle as the days grow short and dark: you feel less than your best so you look less than your best, and that recognition only makes you feel still worse. . . But low spirits and drab looks can have a real basis in fact – they're not just psychosomatic symptoms of the season. In winter the skin retains up to 20 per cent less moisture but our bodies retain twice as much fluid and we eat more 'fuel' food or carbohydrates. The upshot is that toxins build up along with the heavier food and shows up in sluggish skin.

BRACE UP To counteract the effects of winter winds and wet, you should, at least occasionally, meet them head on. Resist the urge to hibernate in front of the video, take bracing walks whenever possible to stimulate the circulation and work off your stodgier diet. Cheeks flushed from a constitutional in the park do you more credit than those reddened by huddling over the radiator.

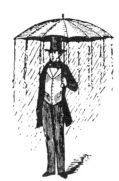

Blow the cobwebs away but don't let a chill wind do you any unnecessary damage. You must use a moisturizer now more then ever – and remember the neck areas as well as the face, for woolly scarves wound round can set up soreness and scratchiness between chin and chest. Don't come rushing in from the cold to steam in a room of the opposite extreme – it's certain to give you a red nose as the blood rushes to heat the coldest extremities. Keep a lipsalve handy and use it regularly to prevent sore, chapped lips.

PISTE OFF

There's no business like snow business, so an increasing number of winter sporters maintain. As a skier you're going out into extreme weather conditions: biting cold winds and a high intensity of sunlight. Either way your skin is likely to dry up and needs protection. Don't ignore the sound snow skin sense that prompts even hardy veterans of national ski teams to wear a sun cream of high protective factor – six, seven or eight depending on your natural skin type. Ears, forehead and nose can get burned quite badly if you don't take precautions. Take plenty of moisturizer with you.

NONE OF YOUR LIP! Lips also get very dried up and chapped. In the sun they may blister; in the wind dry cracks can open up and bleed. To prevent this you're advised not only to arm yourself with your usual lipsalve but to scour chemists and ski shops for lipscreen creams which, like sun creams, are made in different factors.

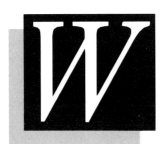

OLE RED EYES Think ahead to eye protection at the planning stage of your skiing holiday. Very strong ultraviolet rays reflect off the snow and these can burn your eyes – even through cheap plastic sunspecs. The whites of your eyes may go very red, and could lead to temporary snow blindness, so it's important to invest in really good quality ski sunglasses available from specialist ski shops or sports stores. The French firm Vuarnet make good glasses, as does the Austrian company Carrera and US companies Scott and Uvex.

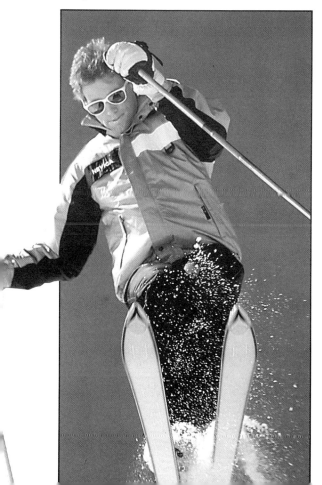

A FACE IN THE SUN

Mad dogs and Englishmen now know better than to go out in the midday sun. Half a century of competitive broiling has given way to dire warnings of skin cancer and ageing wrinkles that result from too much tanning. It turns out that the Victorians who favoured pale and interesting skins were right all along. Bring back the parasol and the panama boater. All is forgiven.

TRUTH ABOUT THE TAN Contrary to popular misconception a tan is not a superficial reward for lying prone on a sunwashed beach for 20 minutes the first day, 30 the next and then some. It is not a splash of becoming colour bestowed by nature as a means of attracting the opposite sex in a Marbella disco. A tan is, in fact, the skin's defensive response against further damage. Melanin, appearing as brown pigment, is activated to rise to the skin surface and prevent further burning by UVB, the middle-range ultraviolet sunlight.

The sad sizzling news is that even after you stop burning the sun is working its subversive ageing mischief, by stimulating new skin cell production that thickens up your skin and lends that leathery look to eternal beach bums. Combined UVA and UVB rays are also doing their worst for future wrinkles, as they damage collagen, DNA and elastin, on whose continued buoyancy good skin depends.

Fair-skinned sunbathers are likely to suffer far more damage than olive or dark skinned members of the population: their skins lack melanin protection. Black skins, and black skins alone, can withstand the heat of the sun without added artificial protection.

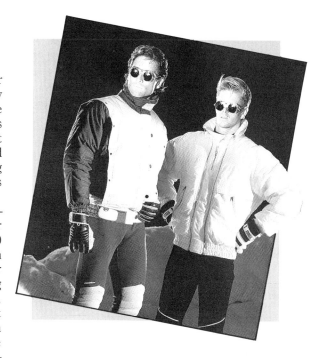

TAKING THE HEAT OUT OF HOLIDAYS Every cloud has its silver lining: two or three weeks only besporting yourself on a sun-kissed beach should not skin you alive. A vast market place of sun-screen and other tanning preparations is yours to make use of, and by buying wisely (you'll need at least two tubes or bottles of cream for a fortnight away – don't scrimp) and applying your purchases liberally before settling back on the beach, you should tan without trouble. Sun-screen preparations are now sold with an SPF (sun protection factor) grading: usually from 2–20. You should start your holiday using a preparation with a high protection factor (above 6) or by using an old-fashioned unglamorous, but highly effective zinc oxide paste bought from your local chemist. If you want to have the appearance of tanning without the risk, then take advantage of the preparations which tint whilst protecting you.

Don't let the sun catch you crying

Do be particularly careful to work up your time in the sun gradually.

Don't lie out in local 'siesta' hours when the sun is at its strongest.

If you do burn, a cut lemon squeezed over the sore areas brings relief. So too, it's claimed, does a capsule of vitamin E broken over the skin so that its oils can soothe and heal.

Be warned that wind and water may give a false impression of keeping you cool: you could still be burning, even if you don't feel it at the time.

Every time you leave the beach have a shower, or wash your face in cool water. Salt sea water and sand could irritate your skin later.

Don't be mean with the moisturizer.

Wear good sunglasses – it is a shame if your even face tan is spotted with two white rings around the eyes. But better pale peepers today than dried prunes in coming years.

Rubbing in baby oil each night after showering or bathing helps to keep your sunned skin supple.

style

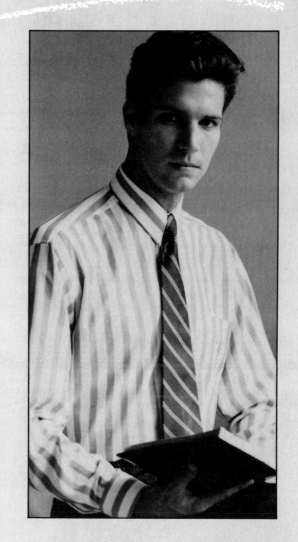

Chic to chic

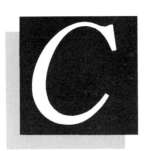

Anatole France once said that if he came back 100 years after his death and could have just one book, he would opt for a fashion magazine because it would tell him the way that people lived. Today a time traveller would find that men have rediscovered their historic interest in clothes. No longer is it thought smart to be scruffy, nowadays it's chic to be chic. Which leaves anyone who has been using the lived-in look as a cover for *laissez-faire*, desperate for a bit of *savoir-faire*.

> *"Whenever two people meet there are really six people present. There is each man as he sees himself, each man as the other person sees him, and each man as he really is."* William James

TOP DRAWER OR BEDROOM FLOOR?

Some men are born knowing exactly how to fold a pocket handkerchief, while nanny struggles to fold the terry nappies. This breed has no trouble tying a proper bow tie or selecting the appropriate attire for every occasion. You can bet there will be at least one of them, all sang-froid and Savile Row, among fellow applicants at any job interview. There he sits, so well-suited for the job, exuding confidence, while lesser mortals contemplate slashing their wrists on the razor-sharp creases of his impeccable trousers.

There is a definite art to looking the part, and with an economic climate that calls for thermal underwear it has never been more important to learn it, yet lots of men remain woefully unbriefed. They often stay that way out of insecurity, opting out rather than sorting out their appearance. These are the men who pretend that the out-of-the-laundry-basket look is a deliberate choice of style and that looking a mess is macho. In fact, looking a mess is merely tacky and unlikely to be tolerated at a time when formal clothes are turning back to traditional classic styles and even casual wear is getting smarter.

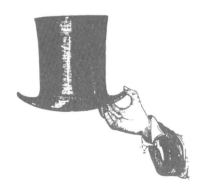

The gap between the well-dressed and the dog-eared is widening and no one really wants to be mistaken for one of the caterers when turning up at a wedding. Anyone who has caught sight of himself in a store window, resolved to do something about his appearance and then chickened out because he didn't know where to start should not despair: polishing up a tarnished image doesn't take all that much elbow grease.

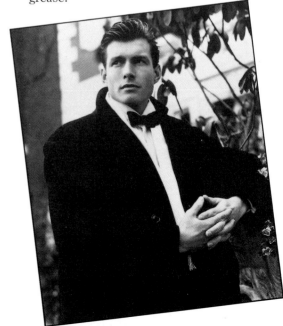

Hot under the collar

Smartening up often requires less effort and discomfort than covering up. We all know someone who spends half their life trying to keep their slovenliness under wraps. He is the master of the layered look, who sits steaming in his jacket to hide the hole in his sweater, worn to conceal the unironed shirt. He seldom buys new shoes because of his holey socks, shrinks from helping old ladies across the road because his underwear wouldn't stand scrutiny if he got involved in an accident, and can't accept any invitation without a last-minute trip to the launderette.

This chap is unlikely to become a picture of sartorial elegance, but with a little effort he could look all right instead of all wrong. A prospective employer will judge by appearances and, unless he's a farmer with a pest control problem, he is unlikely to hire a scarecrow. Anyone who has seen *The Wizard of Oz* (and who can have escaped it?) knows that scarecrows are not only scruffy but brainless.

> "*If a man does not dress well in society he cannot be a success.*"
> 'Bertie', Prince of Wales, later Edward VII

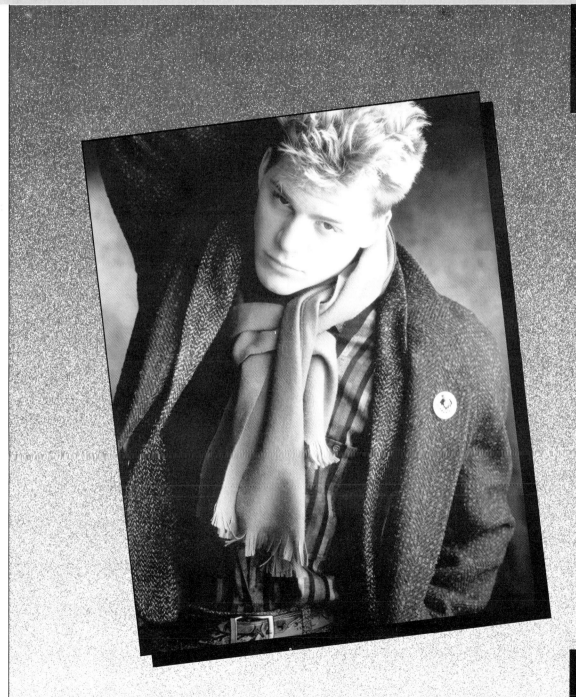

ALL THE NICE GIRLS LOVE A TAILOR

Women too have become more fastidious. These days a smelly old bachelor will probably remain one. Men have lost the sympathy vote, so if they look too lived in they are more likely to be condemned for slum clearance than rescued and renovated. Although girlfriends, wives and mothers still buy a lot of clothes for their men – something like half of all shirts and underpants sold are bought by women – they look before they leap now. The "lovely gifted girls" of Robert Graves' poem are no longer inclined to marry "impossible men. . ./For whose appearance even in City parks/Excuses must be made to casual passers-by."

According to one menswear expert, women tend to "impulse buy" men's clothes. And looking like a collection of someone else's whims hardly gives a chap an impressive image of his own. Nor does being kitted out as if he was still in short trousers do a lot for his self-esteem. There is no sadder sight on a sales floor than a man being "dressed" by his wife. The only reason he endures looking so foolish is because he does not know how to begin to dress himself. It is becoming recognized that real men can manage to buy their own clothes unaided.

Men are spending a higher proportion of their income on clothes and footwear but the average expenditure is still only about £200 a year.

Of course, £200 is nothing when compared with the £100,000 spent on his wardrobe by 'Prinny', the Prince of Wales, in the early 19th century. It is some consolation to know that Beau Brummell didn't consider that such spending had resulted in good taste. As the song says, "You've either got or you haven't got style" and whether you are a royal dandy spending £800 on a greatcoat lined with sables, or the cautious acquirer of your 6.9th pair of socks, you can just as disastrously put your foot in it.

That's The Way The Money Goes

Figures for year up to Oct '86 supplied by Textile Market Studies.

Some 23 million adult males spent a total of around £4,472,000,000 – an average of £200 each.

NUMBER OF GARMENTS. . .		PER MAN . . .
Socks	160 million	6.9 pairs
Shirts	85 million	3.6
Pants	79 million	3.4 pairs
Knitwear	62 million	2.6
Trousers	44 million	1.9 pairs (but includes women's slacks)
Jeans	24 million	1 pair
Ties	22 million	0.95
Jackets	12 million	0.5
Vests	12 million	0.5
Pyjamas	5 million	0.2 pairs
Ready made suits	4½ million	0.19
Anoraks	3 million	0.13
Coats/Raincoats	1½ million	0.06

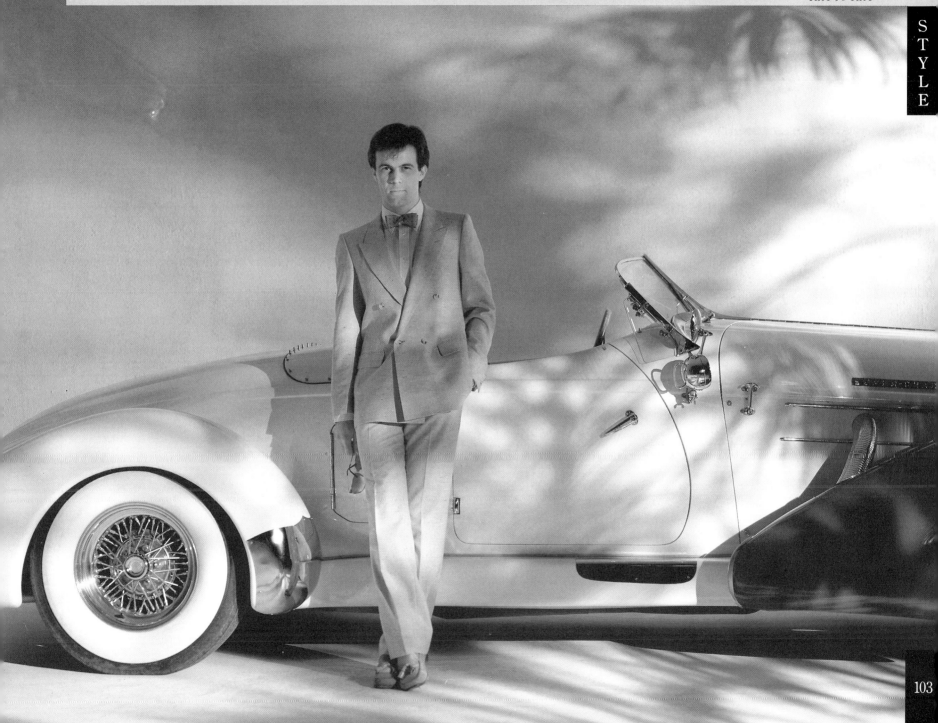

Looking good

STYLE – HOW TO FIND YOURS

A man who hasn't got style is like someone carrying an empty banner – he has got no statement to make and nothing important to say. Style is not encapsulated in the dedicated follower of fashion, slavishly taking up every current craze, nor in Mr Nouveau Riche, thinking he can buy it along with the right designer labels.

There is no way of buying style as a packaged set. You can't send out for it, it has to be home baked, which is why expensive feathers don't necessarily make fine birds. The style of the clothes you wear puts the spotlight on your personality, brings it into focus and broadcasts it. Chainstore or designer clothes, it reflects either the real you or the you you want to project.

> *"The picture of me, the me that is seen is me."*
> D.H. Lawrence

WHO AM I? You are what you wear, and if Oscar Wilde was right "only fools do not judge by appearances". So take a look inside your wardrobe. Imagine a total stranger walking into the room wearing your clothes and ask yourself what you think of him.

The elitist maxim that you can't acquire style is usually bandied about by the sort of arbiters of taste who want to keep lesser men firmly in their place. If a plain Jane can acquire beauty, then a man born without an account at Savile Row, London's elite street of tailoring, or intrinsic exterior designer skills can acquire style. As with everything, if you are not rich or naturally talented you just have to try a bit harder.

Women quite naturally grow up learning to use their eyes and judgment. They learn how to window shop, how to shop around and how to cast a critical eye over the rest of their sex, stealing ideas which can be knit into a look of their own. Men have had less practice, because any young lad who cared too much about his appearance used to be dubbed cissy.

SECOND-HAND POSE Of course all that is changing now. With ten-year-olds developing their own clothes sense anyone can do it. Be warned though, someone who simply poaches fragments of other, classier men and sticks them together is more likely to end up resembling a play school collage than a picture of elegance. It is important that what you buy is right for you. You should feel comfortable about any new ideas and comfortable wearing them. Because you want to project yourself and not merely mimic others make sure you really like your clothes. Then the contents of your wardrobe will conform to your taste and individual style.

If your image calls for a general overhaul it is pointless just going out and buying a few new clothes. Assess what you already have and whether it creates a good picture of you, decide how much of it is worth keeping and what you need to buy to give you a wardrobe well furnished with assets.

> *"Le style est le homme même." (Style is the man.)*
> Comte de Buffon

IF IN DOUBT THROW IT OUT – OVERHAUL YOUR WARDROBE

Try hanging the entire contents of your wardrobe around your bedroom picture rails, lay everything else, down to your socks, on the floor and go over all of it item by item. Be honest and, if necessary, be brutal. Sort everything into three groups – one that is definitely fine, one that will do at a pinch and one that's got to go. Then discard the rejects and replace the remainder, while keeping the best separate from the rest. The clothes that are only passable need replacing as soon as possible. If you've got a very healthy bank balance throw them out with the cast-offs and replace them straight away.

When weighing up old favourites don't cheat and hang on to the shirt with the fraying collar to do the gardening in, it will only sneak back into your life when everything else is in the wash. Don't cram half-a-dozen stretched or shrunken T-shirts back, drop the lot in the bin and buy a couple of new ones.

A wardrobe overflowing with jumble only fools you into thinking that you have got something to wear when you haven't. And beaten up formal wear doesn't downgrade to casual clothes. Bear in mind too that fashions go in 30 year cycles, a long wait if you are saving something outdated waiting for it to make a come-back. In fact, you would probably be better off saving your father's old clothes than your own.

CLOTHES HORSES FOR COURSES

Every occupation has a "uniform", which to a degree will determine the clothes you need for work. You don't have to look the same as everyone else but you do have to look right. The academic has traditionally been seen in sports jackets with elbow patches, wool and cotton mix shirts and corduroys. Doctors, too, when they are not in white coats, opt for a 'folksy' image, a city suit doesn't sit well on a bedside manner.

The advertising man is likely to be all conformist non-conformity and casual chic, while the city whizz-kid sports silk ties and Giorgio Armani suits. Salesmen are usually seen in smart two-piece suits, the price tag and style determined as much by the people he is selling to as by his taste or bank balance – sales technique includes not distancing yourself too far from the customer. Lawyers and senior civil servants, meanwhile, can usually be seen in classic dark pin-stripes, hand-made shirts and sober ties.

> *"Costly thy habit as thy purse can buy,*
> *But not express'd in fancy; rich, not*
> *gaudy: For the apparel oft proclaims*
> *the man."*
> Polonius in Shakespeare's *Hamlet*

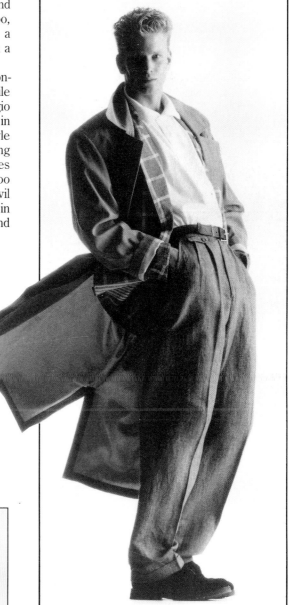

A well-dressed wardrobe should contain:

SUITS
Three or four (if you wear a suit to work)
To include: A good basic grey flannel, a classic stripe, an interesting pattern like Prince of Wales check or herringbone, and a lightweight suit for summer.

JACKETS
For work or smart casual wear
A well-cut blazer (if you're a blazer man), two sports jackets to include: one in grey or black & white, one in blue or the brown/green look.

TROUSERS
To team with smart jackets three or four pairs to include:
A pair of classic flannel twills
Possible upper-crust cavalry
A discreet pattern (like houndstooth)
summer slacks
(As a general rule plain slacks with patterned jackets and vice versa.)

FORMAL EVENING WEAR
(If you attend a lot of formal or dressy functions)
Dinner suit and dress shirt (shawl collars outlast fashion)
And/or black slacks and party jacket (with silk faced lapels) or white tuxedo.

OVERCOAT/RAINCOAT
To cover a suit a classic navy or grey top coat
And/or a Burberry style trench coat.

SHIRTS
You can't have too many shirts to team with suits and sports coats. A minimum of one for each day of the week plus extras for evenings, to include:
Classic whites, other plain colours with contrast collars an option, and traditional stripes, which team with any suit.

TIES
(No tired or stained ties please)
Again you can't have too many, for best effect include: Solid colours, stripes, pattern repeats and dots, which look good with everything, and a bow tie for evening.

106

OFF-DUTY TROUSERS

For casual, casual not smart, casual wear
Two pairs to include: Corduroys, canvas, cotton or denim.

OFF-DUTY SHIRTS

Three or four to include: Checks, dark coloured casual shirts and short-sleeved lightweight, sports or T-shirts for summer.

KNITWEAR

Crewneck, rollneck and V-neck (sleeved and sleeveless) sweaters to team with sports jackets
Traditional hand-knits such as Arran or Fair Isle patterns, trendies can go for fashion knits for casual wear
Cotton or lightweight wool for summer.

CITY SHOES

Three pairs at least to team with smart attire
Classics with leather uppers and soles, including a brogue effect.

OFF-DUTY COAT OR JACKET

For casual or country wear
A winterweight or weather-proof cover-up like a three-quarter length casual jacket
A lightweight jacket or blouson top.

SOCKS AND BOXERS

Enough cotton/cotton blend summer socks and wool/wool blend winter socks to wear with everything
Boxer shorts or cotton slips and a pair of pyjamas for emergency hospital admission. . .

OFF-DUTY SHOES

No city shoes with casual wear please
One pair of soft smart casuals
One deck shoe or sports type shoe
Wellies and specialist sports shoes.

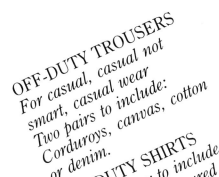

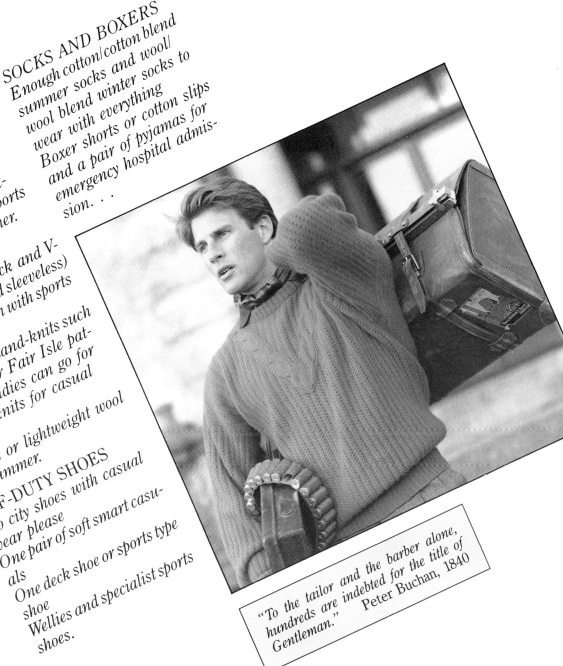

"To the tailor and the barber alone, hundreds are indebted for the title of Gentleman." Peter Buchan, 1840

MOVING UP

If you have decided to take your image up market you may well need to start shopping somewhere new. Men often dislike shopping, seeing it as an unmanly activity and resenting the time spent on it. For most of history, however, it was men who did all the family shopping in the town or city because men did all the travelling. They bought everything from their wives' bonnets to cloth for the clothes of the entire family.

You will never buy wisely if you rush into a shop and grab, neither will your style change a great deal if it is always the same shop. According to one menswear expert, "Men stick with a label and often stay with one store for fifteen years or more until something or someone upsets them." Don't wait for grounds for divorce.

A particular tailor's may have been fine for your father, or right for you when you were 17, but you don't have to stay together for life. Your style can't grow up as you grow older if you never broaden your horizons. So go walkabout – visit a variety of shops simply to consider and price their clothes. You may well find that an elegant two-piece suit in a classy shop costs little more than a very ordinary one elsewhere and that you would be happy to pay the extra.

If you feel particularly sensitive, do your shopping around at the busiest time when you won't be hassled by pushy salesmen or look too conspicuous. Looking like a downbeat man in an up-tempo shop is a sure sign that your image does need smartening up. So don't be put off, you can't spend life unable to go to a decent tailor's because you've got nothing to wear.

MIRROR, MIRROR ON THE WALL

Before you actually buy new clothes take a good look at yourself. You need to know your shape to start to cut a figure so take the blinkers off and confront the real you in a full-length mirror. Once you have determined your faults there are less drastic solutions than major cosmetic surgery, a crash diet or hara-kiri.

A British Clothing Centre survey of around 1000 men gives some idea of the shape and weight of the average man.

JEKYLL YOUR HYDE – ILLUSION DRESSING

If you don't have a standard shaped body, even if it is rather weird, you can always Jekyll your Hyde. The experts call it "illusion dressing". It is a way of emphasizing your assets and disguising your liabilities – in other words cheating. Cheating of this sort has an excellent pedigree. Back in 1784 'Prinny', Prince of Wales, put the royal stamp on high-rise cravats because he wanted to conceal his swollen neck glands.

A mirror will tell you the truth about your problem areas, but so will the clothes you have been wearing if you look at how they have sagged, bagged, stretched or wrinkled. You can ignore your paunch in the mirror but not the paunch in your trousers. Staying with the size you were before you took to the ale or gave up playing football is only going to make you appear portlier, not keep you sylph-like.

> "O wad some Pow'r the giftie gie us
> To see oursels as others see us!
> It wad frae mony a blunder free us
> And foolish notion".   Robert Burns

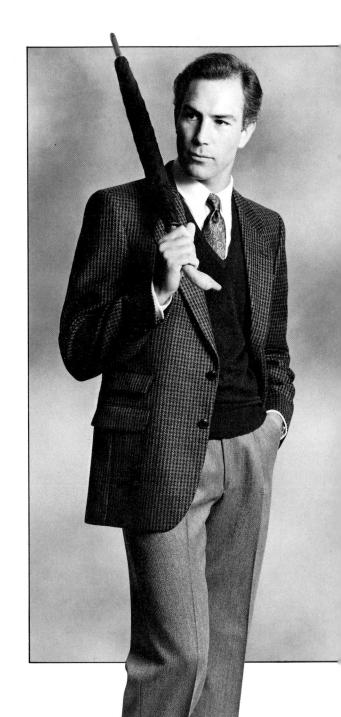

British Clothing Centre Survey

	AGE	AVERAGE SIZE	SIZE RANGE
NECK	Under 26	14.4"	11.8" – 16.9"
		36.7cm	30.0 – 43.0cm
	26+	14.9"	10.2" – 18.5"
		38.0	26.0 – 47.0
CHEST	Under 26	35.8"	29.0" – 45.7"
		91.1	73.8" – 116.2
	26+	37.9"	31.0" – 51.5"
		96.5	78.8 – 130.9
WAIST	Under 26	30.4"	24.9" – 41.4"
		77.3	63.3 – 105.2
	26+	32.7"	26.0" – 48.3"
			66.2 – 122.7
HIP	Under 26	37.1"	32.2" – 48.2"
		94.4	81.9 – 122.6
	26+	38.3"	32.8" – 49.8"
		97.5	83.5 – 126.6
INSIDE LEG	Under 26	32.7"	25.7" – 38.7"
		83.2	65.4 – 98.4
	26+	32.2"	25.3" – 37.8"
		81.9	64.3 – 96.1
WEIGHT	Under 26	156.6lbs	106.7lb – 261.6lb
		71.2	48.5 – 118.9
	26+	166.9lbs	114.8lb – 263.6lb
		75.9	52.2 – 119.8
HEIGHT	Under 26	69.0"	59.7" – 76.3"
		175.4	151.7 – 194.3
	26+	68.4"	59.9" – 75.5"
		173.8	152.2 – 191.8

measurements in inches   lbs
                    cms   kgs

"*The Right Hon. was a tubby little chap who looked as if he had been poured into his clothes and forgotten to say, 'When!'".*   P.G. Wodehouse

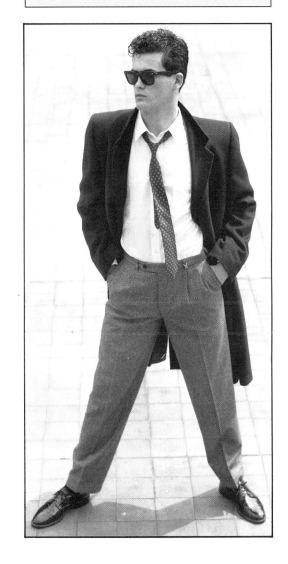

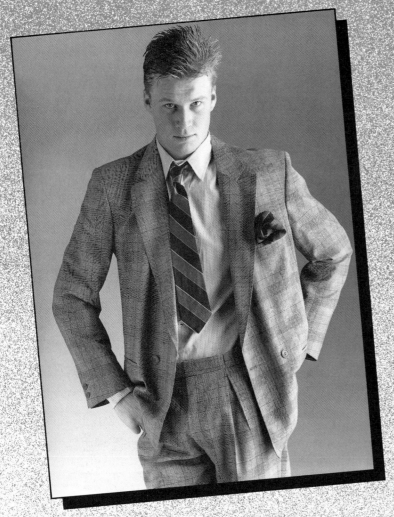

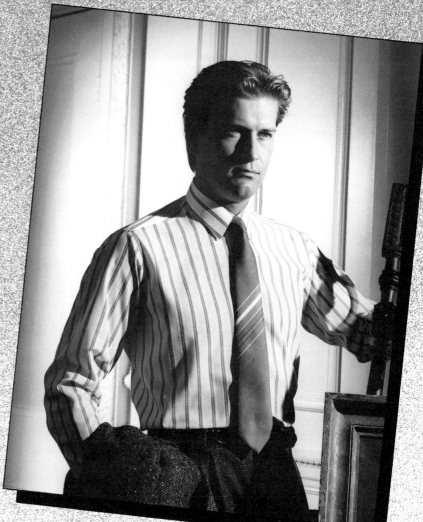

Trousers were not designed to act like corsets on your body, so that it bursts forth once they are unfastened like a self-inflating life-raft. If you go up a size, do the decent thing, and take your trousers along with you. The front pockets on your trousers should lie almost flat against the trousers themselves. If your pockets bulge then your trousers are carrying more stomach than they were made to. Waist fastenings coming adrift and creases across the lap are caused by the same problem, while creasing on thighs and knees means the trouser legs are too tight. Change the size if they are too small in the body, the cut if they are too tight in the leg.

Sticking with the wrong collar size is another common failing. If the points of your shirt collar don't lie flat against the shirt front, if the shirt pulls and wrinkles between collar and chest or your tie doesn't sit neatly inside the collar spread, then you need a larger collar size. And if you look as though you are coming up for air, with your collar forming a V-neck or hanging lop-sided inside your jacket you need a smaller size. A properly fitting collar is one that allows you to insert just one finger between collar and neck.

If you don't want to look like a stuffed shirt check on the fit across your body. When buttons on your shirt front pull or come off and the material gapes between the fastenings and creases across the chest you need a change. You may need a fuller fit in the same brand or a slim fit in another make. Some brands are cut trimmer than others so you need to find the right one for you.

THE BODY SCRUTABLE A man's shoulders are normally broader than his hips. Some men have extremely broad shoulders, however, some have shoulders and hips almost the same size and shape and others are broader in the hip than the shoulders.

A broad shouldered man's shoulders should not jut out beyond the seam in the jacket where the sleeve is sewn in. There should be a smooth line from the top of the shoulder to the bottom of the sleeve. If he wants to give balance below the waist, pocket flaps on jackets and pleated trousers can help. Narrow lapels are best avoided and well-cut double-breasted jackets look good on this shape.

Square or pear shapes benefit from jacket shoulder padding to make more of their shoulders. Hips can be slimmed down by avoiding pleating on trousers and choosing front pockets cut on the slant. Sweaters and shirts with set-in sleeves also add width to the shoulders.

THE LONG AND THE SHORT AND THE TALL A lot of exceedingly tall men are so sensitive about their height that they perpetually sag at the knees and droop at the shoulders, while never giving a thought to the type of clothes that would shrink them visually.

LOOKING SHORTER Patterns like checks look better than plain colours. Vertical stripes, like pin-stripes or corduroy, elongate and are best avoided. Wearing dark sweaters or jackets with lighter coloured slacks reduces height. Trouser turn-ups and a fairly wide belt also help.

Short men too are sensitive about their height and worry about being thought of as little men. At its worst this complex can affect your choice of career – to quote Woody Allen, "I wanted to be an arch-criminal as a child, before I discovered I was too short." But there are better ways than platform soles to add height.

LOOKING TALLER Vertical stripes will give more height, but avoid checks or heavy fabrics, like tweeds, which tend to add width. Too much contrast between top and bottom garments will slice you in half. Blending jacket, trousers and shoes will make you look taller. Trousers without turn-ups are best.

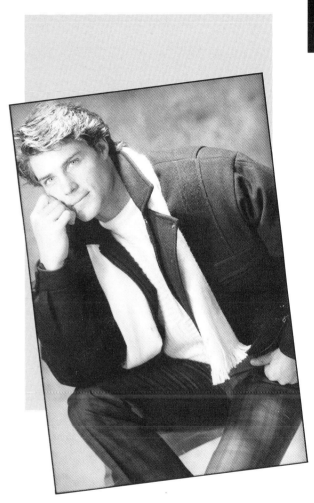

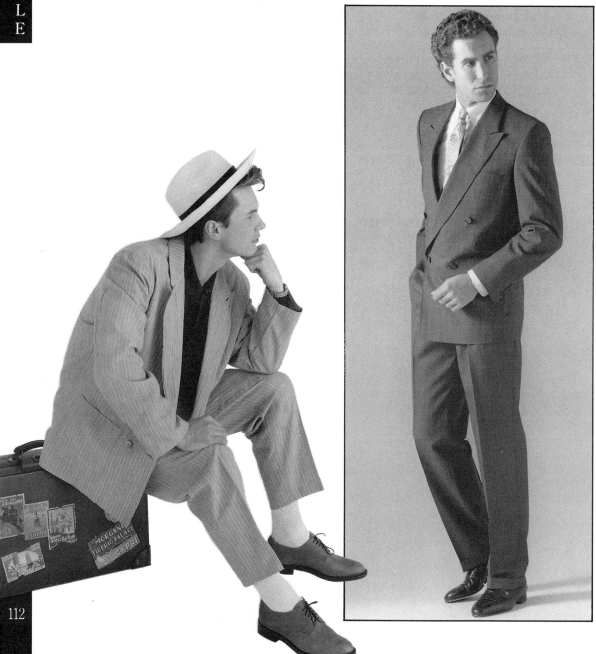

LOOKING SLIMMER Opt for vertical stripes, wool blends or solid colour to look slimmer. Avoid horizontal designs, checks and heavier tweeds, which add bulk.

LOOKING BROADER If you are in danger of being popped into the umbrella stand try shoulder padding and double breasted jackets to fill you out. Checks, heavy fabrics and sweaters with horizontal stripes help too.

TURN-UP FOR THE LOOKS If you are absolutely in proportion your legs make up half your total height. Turns-ups, which should generally be about one and a half inches, can make a long leg look shorter, trouser legs without turn-ups look longer.

WAISTS & STRAYS Standing sideways on to a mirror in belted trousers will give you an idea if your waist is where it ought to be. To lift your waistline match your trouser belt with your trousers, to drop it match your belt with your shirt.

ARMS AND THE MAN If you want your arms to appear longer than they are show a bit more than the customary half an inch of cuff below your jacket sleeve, or if you want to shorten long arms show a bit less than half an inch.

> *"If a man's professional status and identity are important to him, he always needs to look fresh and dynamic, which calls for a wardrobe of at least four suits."*
> John Jelieneck, formal wear buyer,
> Principles for Men

Women have been fooling everyone for years by dressing up their best features while playing down their worst, and sensible men do the same. You want to be remembered but not as the fat man in trendy tartan trousers.

Men's Sizes in the United Kingdom

Chart Shows Imperial and Metric Dimensions for Men's Outerwear
Chart compiled by the Federation of Clothing Designers and Executives

MEN'S REGULAR SIZES (5 FT 8 IN. TO 5 FT 10 IN.)

CHEST

inches	34	35	36	37	38	39	40	41	42	43	44	45	46	47	48
centimetres	86	89	91	94	97	99	102	104	107	109	112	114	117	119	122

TROUSER	29	30	31	32	33	34	35	36	37½	39	40	41	42	43	44
WAIST	74	76	79	81	84	86	89	91	95	99	102	104	107	109	112

INSIDE	30	30½	31	31	31	31	31	31	31	31	31	30½	30½	30½	30½
LEG	76	78	79	79	79	79	79	79	79	79	79	78	78	78	78

MEN'S LONG SIZES (5 FT 11 IN. TO 6 FT 1 IN.)

CHEST

inches	34	35	36	37	38	39	40	41	42	43	44	45	46	47	48
centimetres	86	89	91	94	97	99	102	104	107	109	112	114	117	119	122

TROUSER	29	30	31	32	33	34	35	36	37½	39	40	41	42	43	44
WAIST	74	76	79	81	84	86	89	91	95	99	102	104	107	109	112

INSIDE	31½	32	32½	32½	32½	32½	32½	32½	32½	32½	32½	32	32	32	32
LEG	80	81	83	83	83	83	83	83	83	83	83	81	81	81	81

MEN'S SHORT SIZES (5 FT 5 IN. TO 5 FT 7 IN.)

CHEST

inches	34	35	36	37	38	39	40	41	42	43	44	45	46	47	48
centimetres	86	89	91	94	97	99	102	104	107	109	112	114	117	119	122

TROUSER	29	30	31	32	33	34	35	36	37½	39	40	41	42	43	44
WAIST	74	76	79	81	84	86	89	91	95	99	102	104	107	109	112

INSIDE	28½	29	29½	29½	29½	29½	29½	29½	29½	29½	29½	29	29	29	29
LEG	72	74	75	75	75	75	75	75	75	75	75	74	74	74	74

On parade

> "It's the sort of suit you walk into a tailor's in and ask for the cheapest suit in the shop and he says 'you're wearing it'."
> Trevor Griffiths
> *The Comedians*

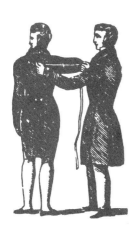

SUIT YOURSELF

It has been said that a suit should cost at least a week's wages, so it follows that if it takes that much earning a suit should do more for you than simply cover your body and keep out the cold.

Some four and a half million ready made suits are sold each year in the UK. Viewed one way that's not an awful lot of suits (something like 0.19 of a suit per man per year). But looked at in another it is four and a half million possible mistakes.

A suit will be the biggest investment in your wardrobe. If you choose a style that does not date and look after it properly it could be around your life for anything up to a decade, so it pays to get it right when you buy.

WELL SUITED Choosing a suit is rather like choosing a wife: you are going to be together for a long time so you need to be sure it's the real thing. If you are buying one off-the-peg you need to spend time selecting and sizing up the suits on offer.

Don't simply stand in front of a rail of suits in your size trying to weigh them up by the look of their left sleeves. That is like searching for a favourite author by contemplating the binding on the book spines in the library. Get a number of suits down off the rail and look at them properly.

Take your time and ignore the salesman who is intent on rushing you into a decision, telling you every time you slip a jacket on, "It's really you, sir." He has got to sell it not wear it, you are the one who will have to pay for

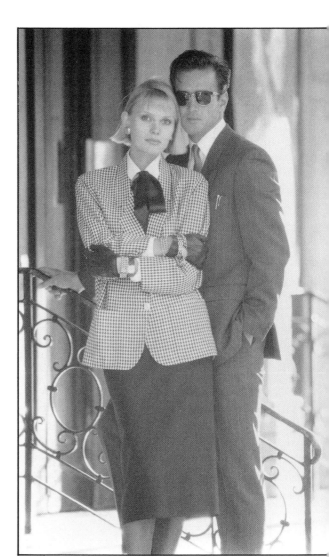

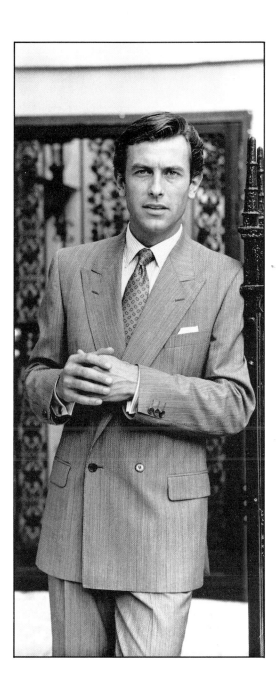

your mistakes. There is nothing worse than having to wear a suit for ages when you realized in the first week that it didn't look good on you.

ACCORDING TO YOUR CLOTH Before you get as far as trying on your suit you will have to make a choice about the type of fabric. Natural fibres have become ever more popular, the clothing equivalent of wholemeal bread. There is a definite move back to nature and away from the man-made. Pure new wool is a label greatly in favour today, but every cloth has its advantages and drawbacks so use your judgment, don't just take to wool like sheep.

The first thing to remember about fabric is that it isn't a case of the more you spend the longer it will last. In fact, it is quite the reverse. Durability is not the name of the game, what you pay for is quality, not mileage. Some men wonder why their expensive suit only lasted half as long as a cheaper one and are left feeling cheated. But the cheaper the fabric, the coarser the cloth and the longer it will last.

The classic British three-piece suit of coat, waistcoat and trousers or knee-breeches is about 380 years old. The two-piece suit is 130.

"A good suit should last about ten years if you look after it properly. If you don't go over the top with the cut you should be able to wear the suit you buy today in ten years time." Tommy Nutter

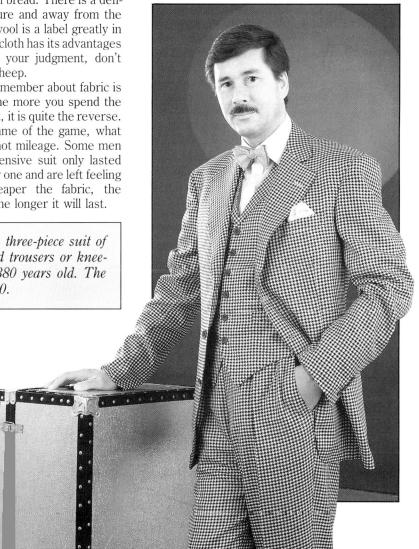

> *Cashmere is the fine, downy wool at the roots of the hair of Kashmir goats, which have to be dehaired by constant combing. Much of it comes from China.*

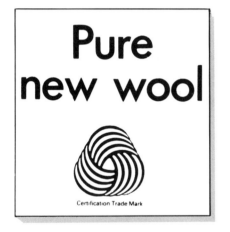

Pure new wool

Certification Trade Mark

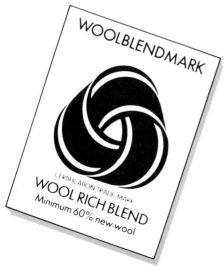

WOOLBLENDMARK

CERTIFICATION TRADE MARK
WOOL RICH BLEND
Minimum 60% new wool

SHEEP FROM THE GOATS The most expensive fabric is pure cashmere, a suit made in this will cost in excess of £1,000. This gentleman's 'mink' is a luxury fibre, which has to be treated with care. Both light and warm it is chosen for its luxury, scarcity or snob value. It is hardly an ideal fabric for a suit, which is why one Savile Row tailor says he would never recommend it to his customers. Another top people's tailor explained, however, "It does feel wonderful next to the skin, a lady would undoubtedly prefer to snuggle up next to a cashmere cloth".

After cashmere in price comes another costly cloth called Lumbs Super Hundred or Golden Bale. This is the aristocrat of the wool world, being wool taken from the very best part of the sheep (from under the neck where the elements haven't reached), and spun finer. Warm and light, it feels rather similar to cashmere to the touch.

POLY, WOOLLY, DOODLE Assuming that you are not going to be tripping off to work in the very finest of cloths, the top end of the price range for you will mean 'pure' wool. This is a soft, comfortable fabric but it does crease, doesn't hold its shape as well as a blended fabric and it needs 'resting' – a suit in pure wool should not be worn every day. Someone who sits in a car for much of their working life, as some salesmen do, would look pretty creased in an all wool suit.

Wool and mohair mix is a combination which used to be popular but has fallen from favour. Wool gives the mohair a softer feel, while mohair cuts down on creasing and helps keep a suit in shape. The drawbacks, however, are that this fabric tends to go shiny and if pressed or dry cleaned too often it can crack along the crease.

Today's popular blend is wool and polyester. At the most expensive end of the price range comes 'Wool Rich', which has to be a minimum

of 60 per cent wool. This fabric can bear the 'Woolblend Mark', not to be confused with the very similar 'Wool Mark', which labels pure wool cloth.

At the cheapest end comes 'Poly Rich', a blend of more polyester than wool. The polyester in a cloth helps a suit hold its shape and resists creasing. Generally speaking, the higher the wool content the higher the price and the softer the fabric, the higher the polyester content the coarser the fabric, but the more durable and crease free.

It is a question of deciding which cloth suits your purpose. David McCall, menswear marketing manager of a leading chainstore, explains, "A pure new wool suit at the top end of our price range will be a beautifully milled fabric, it is that much finer than a wool/polyester or polyester/wool blend so it won't take the same degree of bashing, won't last as long and needs to be more carefully maintained and worn. With fabrics it is very much horses for courses."

NOT SO PRETTY POLY The cheapest and most durable suit cloth is 100 per cent polyester. This holds the trouser creases and the shape of the suit, doesn't wrinkle and is often washable. It is, however, a very stiff, coarse cloth and with wool growing in popularity 100 per cent polyester is increasingly thought of as very down market in suits.

Many companies don't market polyester suits. As one buyer put it, "Who wants to walk about in a cardboard box?" One leading high street chain has dropped 100 per cent poly suits, both their 'classic' and 'fashion' suits come in wool or woolblend. Only their 'mixers', a more trendy, suit-at-a-price for younger customers come in cheaper mixed fibres.

There are suits made in other cloths: washable cotton suits, cotton and linen, even silk. But pure wool, a mixture of wool and polyester, or 100 per cent polyester are the fabrics you will find hanging on the ready-made rails.

PLAIN OR FANCY Having chosen a type of fabric you will then be deciding the colour and pattern you want it to come in. Brown is less popular in suits today, the favourites are blue and grey, lighter shades in summer and darker in winter. If you only keep a suit for formal occasions and don't wear one for work, a classic grey flannel is smart and safe. It will dress up for a dinner or tone down for a memorial service or funeral.

You may decide to go for a solid colour or a colour textured into a subtle pattern by using either a stripe or herringbone effect in the same colour – a self stripe.

If you favour checks beware, they look best on a big man and need choosing with care. In a suit a subtle blend of colours is preferable to a more dramatic colour combination – you don't want your business suit to look as if it escaped from a travelling circus.

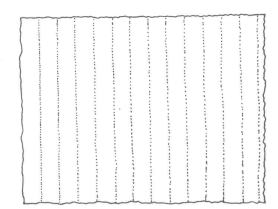

Stripes are extremely popular, particularly pinstripes, which come in differing designs and spacings, anything from one-sixteenth of an inch to one inch apart. Chalk stripes are a smart alternative in a city suit – here stripes are slightly broader and resemble the lines made with a tailor's chalk.

Fancy stripes too are making a comeback after a fairly conservative phase. Here you have coloured stripes on a contrast background, red on grey or a different shade of blue on blue, instead of the usual white of the pinstripe. These candy stripes can look very attractive if they are not too lively. Generally speaking, if you can see a stripe across a crowded room the effect will be less than enchanting, you will either look like a goon or a gangster.

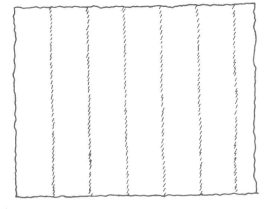

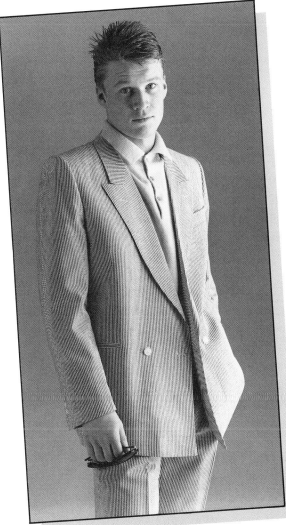

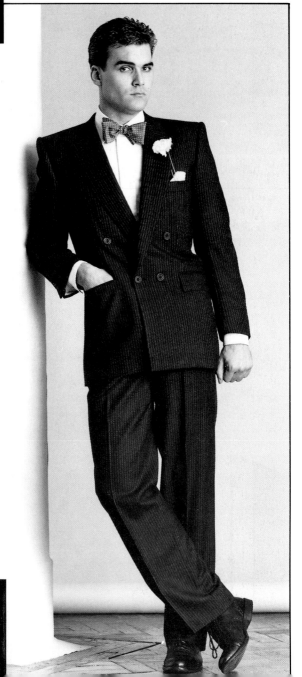

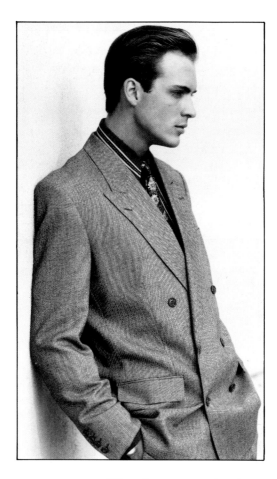

CUTTING A DASH When it comes to the shape of a suit the ones you see will be of classic European cut, or variations on that theme reflecting current fashion. The European suit is quite slim fitting. It has square shoulders and a nipped in waist, and currently double-breasted styles are very popular. The Americans favour a squarer style based on their original "sack suit", a fuller cut with unpadded shoulders.

If you want your suit to last, a 'safe' lapel width is around three inches. Lapels used to be one of the main features that dated a suit. Nowadays, however, lapel widths are as much a matter of taste as fashion. Wider lapels are stylish, especially on a double-breasted jacket worn by a man with broad shoulders. Today's freedom of expression means that you can get away with most things if they are a deliberate choice and not simply a sign that you have been left behind. Even along Savile Row you will find suits being made with lapels varying from two and a half to four and a half inches in width.

Italian suits are still seen as the best. According to one menswear boss, "In creative terms they are still the leaders in fabric and construction." The country of origin isn't as important as it used to be, however, with first-rate suits coming from many more countries, in particular in the EEC. West Germany and Sweden, for example, now produce suits to compete with Italian ones. Most of our suits are imported, something like 70 per cent of all suits sold in the UK coming from overseas, mostly from Romania, Italy, Hong Kong, Portugal, West Germany, Yugoslavia and Hungary.

FITS AND STARTS When finding your correct size in an off-the-peg suit you always have to get the jacket right first because trousers are so much easier to alter. But at last the tailoring trade has stumbled on a whole new idea – suits that actually fit! Men no longer have to go through life with a complex over their inside leg measurement. If your inside leg comes outside the standard sizing for jacket and trousers combined you can now buy the two items separately.

The mix and match suit was pioneered by a leading chainstore in the early seventies and now other companies have followed their lead, many now selling suit jackets and trousers separately.

When trying on there are some simple rules you can follow:

Does it fit?

SLEEVES
Should just cover your wrist bone, while allowing half an inch of shirt cuff to show (wear one of your normal shirts when trying on suits).

COLLARS
Should hug the back of your neck, while allowing a bit of shirt collar to show above them.

CHEST
Should allow movement. Check by doing the jacket up and reaching forward. The jacket should lie flat on your chest with no gaping lapels.

JACKET LENGTH
Jackets should cover your bottom without hanging down too far if you don't want the Tweedledum or Teddy boy look. Tailors used to say that when your arms hang straight by your sides the hem of a jacket should sit in your curled fingers.

VENTS
Should not pull open when you stand up straight.

SHOULDERS
Should have an unbroken line – no parrot's perch unless you are auditioning for Long John Silver in panto.

TROUSERS
Ensure that the rise (distance between crotch and waist) is comfortable and that the seat fits properly. Even if 'baggy' trousers are in vogue, the sag is not supposed to be on the bum.

TROUSER CREASES
Should be visible from a point where the front pockets end all the way down (horizontal lines mean trousers are too tight) and should fall centred over the middle toe, as long as your legs aren't of the knock-kneed or bow-legged variety.

TROUSER HEM
Should clear the heel of your shoe and break on the front. Avoid the concertina effect, which makes you look as if you have been dropped from a great height and hit solid concrete, and the cut-off-short variety, which gives the impression that you bought the trousers before you stopped growing. You need a little more length than it takes to just touch your shoe tops.

ENGLISH AS SHE IS BESPOKE If you want a suit that really fits you can always opt for made-to-measure. You will, of course, pay more if you go for bespoke. How much more depends on the tailor, the cloth, and just how made-to-measure the suit really is. A middle of the range suit will probably cost around an extra 60 per cent for made-to-measure than for off-the-peg. This will be made from a stock pattern which is adjusted to your measurement. The upper-crust when they want to be every inch a gentleman saunter along to London's Savile Row, where the perfect fit is achieved by making an individual pattern for each customer's suit, which will normally be made on the premises. If you are a high society swell rather than a High Street shopper your two-piece tailor-made Savile Row suit can run to well in excess of £1,000.

Tommy Nutter, from No 19, has a clientele which includes members of the Royal Family, Hardy Amies, Lord and Lady Montagu of Beaulieu, the Saatchi brothers and Sir Roy Strong. The Savile Row bespoke service, he says, means, "You hardly feel as if you are wearing a suit because you do get the perfect fit."

Not only does a suit from 'The Row' have the right pedigree to pad along the corridors of power, a discerning eye can even spot the kennel it came from. Each house has its subtleties of style – one favours wider lapels, another a more shaped cut to the jacket. The discerning will know the difference between a Huntsman suit and an Anderson & Sheppard.

Enfant innovateur of the Savile Row scene, Tommy Nutter makes suits "with an outline which is a little more up to date". They are based on a classic cut but with a wider, squarer shoulder, very close hips on the jacket but no flare and no vents. Deeply pleated trousers, which are fairly wide but taper at the bottom and often come with turn-ups. He is also into fancy waistcoats.

The fact that the waistcoat is becoming a thing of the past is, in fact, more a matter of economics than a statement of acceptable style. It is not that waistcoats are 'out' but that three-piece suits cost something like an extra 10 per cent to 15 per cent more than two-piece. As for fancy waistcoats, you need to be either very confident in your style or a snooker player to get away with them.

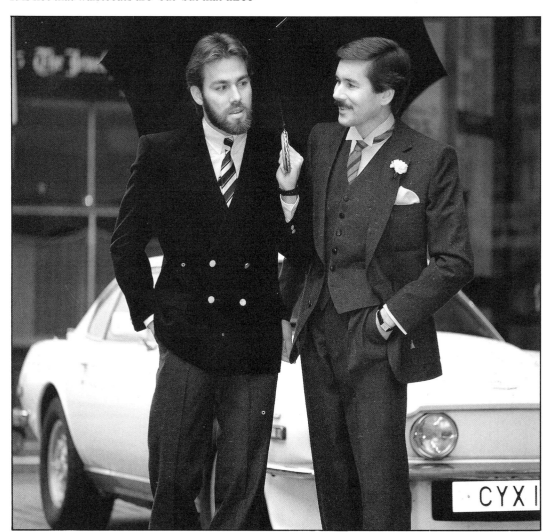

GETTING SHIRTY

Burlington Bertie may have managed without a single shirt but today's Mr Average buys 3.6 a year. His preference is for plain colours – white comes top of the list, followed by blue and then cream. Stripes account for around 30 per cent of all shirts sold. But on the top layers of the socio-economic strata stripes are *de rigueur* – the Bengal stripe being essential to the city gent uniform.

The shirt was born in the 15th century and grew buttons 100 years later. Sadly, some men look as if theirs have escaped from a costume museum and lost their buttons along the way. It is little use carefully selecting a suit for going up in the world if you reduce it to the ranks with a shabby old shirt. Don't imagine that no one will notice if you relocate the collar crease to hide the frayed bit – your tie will only stick out under the collar. Don't kid yourself that a tie will act as stand-in for a missing top button. Most of all, don't pretend that your greying or yellowed shirt will pass for white; you will only end up standing next to Mr Clean, whereupon everyone will know just whose mum has not been using Persil.

Avoid too 'busy' shirts or those that come courtesy of Technicolor. No little motifs and no combination of every kind of stripe crammed into one shirt front, in daringly dynamic colours like Dijon *moutarde* or Co-op green. Bold stripes of the classic Bengal, one-eighth-of-an-inch white/one-eight-of-an-inch colour, variety look very distinguished. The ones to keep away from are those that leave anyone looking at you reaching for the vertical hold.

Be careful too when buying 'lively' colours; they may look great in the shop under artificial lighting but they tend to be like the oil paintings brought back off continental holidays – not quite the same when you get them home.

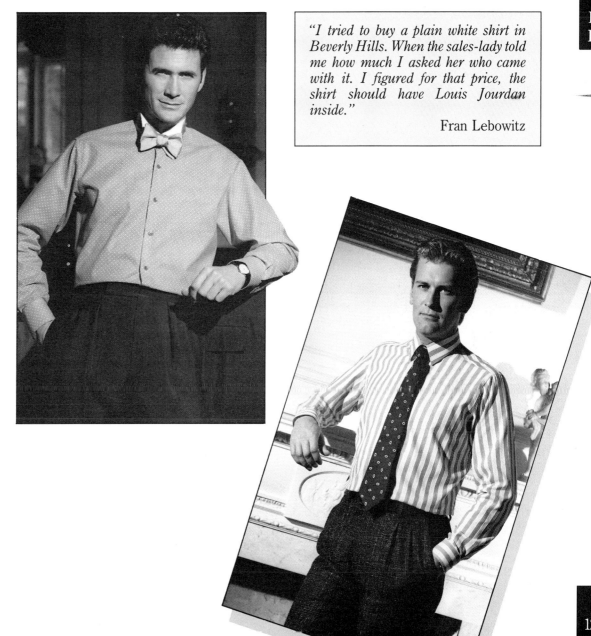

> "I tried to buy a plain white shirt in Beverly Hills. When the sales-lady told me how much I asked her who came with it. I figured for that price, the shirt should have Louis Jourdan inside."
>
> Fran Lebowitz

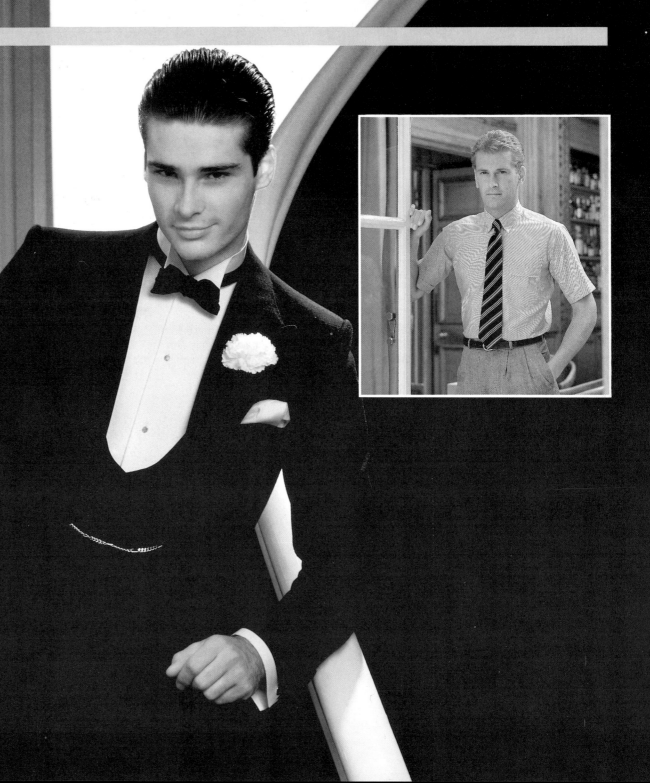

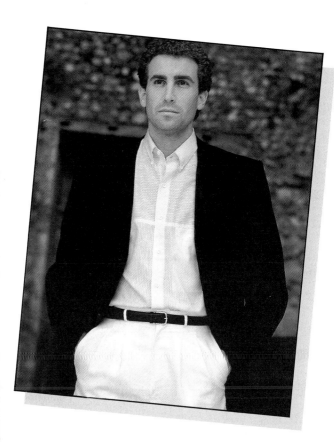

ANYTHING IN A SHIRT A girl might not choose a man simply for his taste in shirts, but she is less likely to fall for someone who wears period-piece collars, or who can't reverse his Granada *Ghia* into a parking space because his tailored fit is too tight. The right kind of shirt is definitely a turn-on. Said Diahann Carroll of Harry Belafonte, "From the top of his head right down that white shirt, he's the most beautiful man I ever set eyes on." Can you imagine her saying, "right down that lilac and plum striped shirt"?

Women actually buy about 48 per cent of all shirts purchased, and in the run up to Christmas it increases to something like 70 per cent. They don't buy as many of the most pricy shirts, probably because these are usually sold in specialist menswear stores, where women don't shop, and probably because better-heeled men tend to dress themselves.

Your mum's and Aunty Ethel's Christmas presents should not, in any case, be the mainstay of your shirt wardrobe. Living in those safe, old-fashioned poly-cottons, which came boxed with toning ties, spells death to individuality and style.

WICKABILITY, THAT'S THE BEAUTY OF COTTON
The swing to a natural fibre diet in menswear means that now the pure wool suit is quite likely to be worn with the all-cotton shirt. The great thing about cotton is that it breathes. Or to put it technically it has a high degree of 'wickability'. A wick is a measure of yarn and wickability is the ability of the cloth to transfer moisture from one side of it to the other. Cotton lets perspiration through to dry off, man-made fibres trap the moisture inside. So if no one wants to stand next to you in a heatwave, consider switching to a cotton shirt.

There has been a big increase in sales of all-cotton shirts and they are certainly more pleasant to wear than those with a high polyester content. But, as ever, there are drawbacks – higher prices, extra time spent ironing and more creases by the end of the day – makes you wonder why God didn't make sheep and cotton bolls crease-resistant.

The fact that they can be difficult to iron stops a lot of people buying cotton shirts. A leading British manufacturer, Van Heusen, claim to have solved the problem with an "easy iron", all-cotton shirt with a special finish, made, says their man coming over all Colonel Saunders, to a "secret formula", and looking extra good.

For the man who shops at the exclusive end of the market, ease of ironing is hardly a consideration. Mr Paul Cuss, with the air of a man whose firm, Turnbull and Asser of Jermyn Street, London, has been bespoke shirtmaker to the gentry for 100 years, explains "A man who owns a Ford may well tinker with it himself. A man who owns a Rolls-Royce has someone to do it for him."

Most of the 500 bespoke and 2000 ready-made shirts made in Turnbull & Asser's workrooms each week come in exclusively designed twofold cotton poplin cloth, the rest come in silk. Initials, or coronets for the peerage, can be hand embroidered on the left-hand side, and boxer shorts, pyjamas and dressing gowns are available in the same shirting materials. The finest silk Turnbull & Asser shirts cost around the same as a decent wool suit for Mr Average. Their cheapest cotton bespoke shirts cost about four times as much as an all-cotton shirt from a bespoke chainstore.

Such shirts are usually found under suits and come with collar bones, double cuffs and good long tails. The man who can afford them does not have his shirt tail hanging out and to him polyester, like formica, is an anathema.

In less elevated circles various blends of polyester and cotton are the norm. Usually the cheaper the shirt the higher the polyester content. If you want comfort without buying all-cotton, a mix of something like 70 per cent cotton to 30 per cent polyester would be a good compromise. Anything that is more than 50 per cent cotton is termed 'cotton rich'. You should find the proportions of the blend labelled on the collar.

GETTING COLLARED There is one rule with collar fads – if you are not sure about a current look, play safe and stick to the standard medium point variety, which always looks good with a city suit. We can only be grateful for the passing of some collar types, the little rounded collar, refugee from the Humpty Dumpty page of a nursery rhyme book, the pinned collar, accidentally shot with that nasty piece of metal.

Some of us hope that the currently popular, cut-away full-spread collar will soon rest in peace too – it should never be worn by a full-faced man or with a narrow tie knot.

Collars with longer than standard points are still around but dated now. The only other acceptable choice is the button-down variety, which can wrinkle if your tie is fairly wide and which some scruffs leave unbuttoned to accommodate their ties. At the chic end of the collar range comes the wing collar, popular now for formal morning or evening wear and extremely fetching.

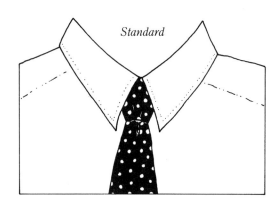

Standard

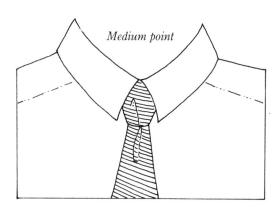

Medium point

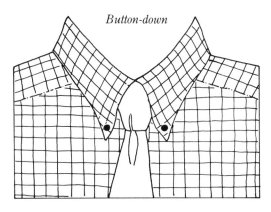

Button-down

FIT FOR ACTION Your shirt should never feel like a strait-jacket and, following the Japanese over-sized look, shirtmakers are producing a more comfortably shaped shirt. Today's shirts are 'shaped' rather than 'tailored' as in the past. Neither tight nor baggy they have more space around the sleeve head to enable wearers to move freely. Branded shirts usually come in standard, shaped fits and full-bodied. Some makes are cut more generously, some have slightly longer sleeves. Shop around and ask advice in the shop to find the fit you need. Normally shirts with 14 and a half – 15 and a half inch collar have 34 inch sleeves, 16 inch collars and above have 35 inch sleeves. If you have long arms one or two companies produce a longer sleeved shirt.

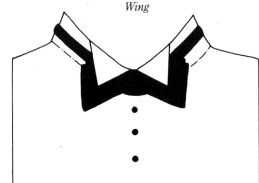

Wing

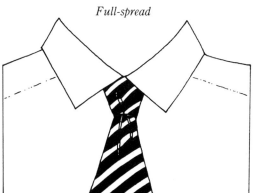

Full-spread

TOP DRESSING

Having found your stylish suit and shirt resist the temptation at all costs to wear a weekend casual coat over the top on a cold day. Those three-quarter-length sheepskins which, once worn for a while, look as if their owners are still inside after they have been taken off, are best left to second-hand car salesmen or the chap selling wristwatches on the pavement.

City suits should only be topped by city overcoats, which come predominantly in navy blue but also in medium and charcoal grey. The camel variety are favoured mostly by older men. The proper length is around the knee, but add two inches for a more fashionable look and always wear a suit when trying on an overcoat.

The only acceptable mackintosh is a Burberry, or Burberry-look-alike, trench-coat style mac. Most macs will be protection against a shower but not against a determined downpour. Choose navy at your peril if you are fresh-faced, because you'll only be taken for a truanting schoolboy.

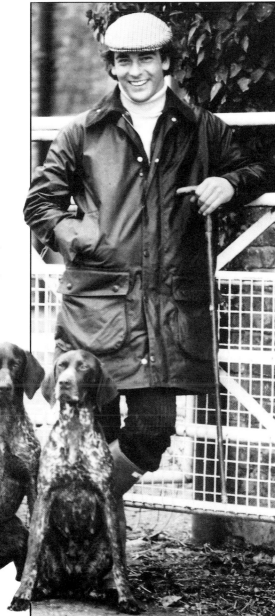

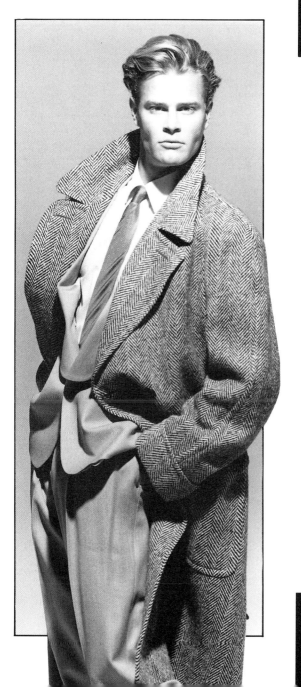

Off duty

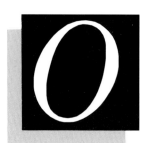

Dressing up

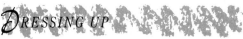

Time was when off-duty meant off-hand in the clothes that you wore. Anything would do – threadbare slacks, holey sweaters. Leisure was *laissez-faire*, dressing up to go out was infra dig. Not anymore. Elegance has expanded to outside office hours and dinner jackets will be worn. There is a theory that when the economy is none too healthy clothes smarten up. A sort of perverse logic says that you can only look down and out when you are not likely to be so. Now the slacks are being pressed and the sweaters come in designer styles. According to the sales manager of the famous hire company, Moss Bros, "More and more people are dressing up and having black tie functions again."

> *"The consciousness of being perfectly dressed may bestow a peace such as religion cannot give."*
> Herbert Spencer

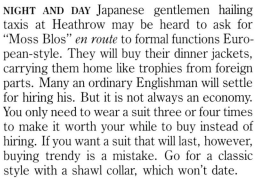

NIGHT AND DAY Japanese gentlemen hailing taxis at Heathrow may be heard to ask for "Moss Blos" *en route* to formal functions European-style. They will buy their dinner jackets, carrying them home like trophies from foreign parts. Many an ordinary Englishman will settle for hiring his. But it is not always an economy. You only need to wear a suit three or four times to make it worth your while to buy instead of hiring. If you want a suit that will last, however, buying trendy is a mistake. Go for a classic style with a shawl collar, which won't date.

"Only buy a very fancy dinner suit if you have got two others in the wardrobe already," says the man from Moss Bros, where a Giorgio Armani evening suit in patterned cloth, with silk toning lapels, costs about three times the price of their classic outfits. Trendy today, you can imagine it hanging alongside all those ghastly braided-lapel dinner jackets in the charity shops tomorrow. The one thing that does date a dinner suit, apart from fashion fads, is the material – barathea, a heavy cloth also used in blazers, has given way now to lighterweight pure new wool.

Most people who wear black tie also wear a cummerbund, meant to cover up the join between trousers and shirt. With double-breasted jackets, which are very popular at present, they are not worn because they would be invisible anyway.

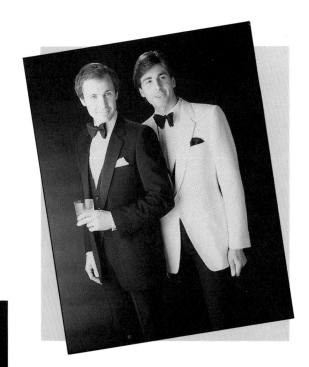

Coloured and variegated cummerbunds, bow ties and pocket handkerchiefs dress up the traditional black and white dinner uniform. Elegant wing collars, sometimes with contrast shirt front, have made a comeback. The smart wing collar shirt, if coloured, comes in beautiful subtle pastels. If the purple shirt is passé so too is the velvet jacket which was often worn by Derek, stalwart MC of the local amateur talent show. White tuxedos, however, have a perennial romantic style. They are usually worn for rather less formal occasions, although in the States they are often worn at weddings.

If you are hiring clothes for either morning wear or evening wear don't leave it until the very last minute. They may be able to kit you out on the spot in London but it is safer to give a couple of weeks notice elsewhere. If you are in any doubt about exactly what to wear for a particular formal occasion, the man who fits you is the expert so don't be afraid to ask his advice. He is the one able to tell you, for example, that morning suits are only worn at the Derby on the day the Derby is actually run because that is when the Queen is present.

Unless you are invited to Royal Ascot the only time you are likely to need morning wear is for a family wedding. Even if this is to be a dressy affair it shouldn't be too uniform. Tail-coats, waistcoats, ties, cravats and collars should not all be an exact match. According to the *Moss Bros Guide To Correct Dress*, "Each male principal and guest should please himself and not be dictated to by the ladies. It is quite wrong for all the men to wear identical outfits."

This does not mean that it is all right for the bride's cousin to act as usher in his motorcycle gear but that there is quite an element of choice within proper morning wear. At no other social occasion would you expect to find half a dozen men with disparate tastes and from two generations dressed identically.

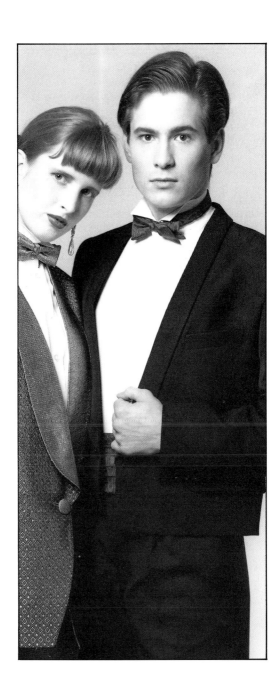

THE BIRTH OF THE TUXEDO

The Prince of Wales (later Edward VII) preferred to wear a short coat, modelled on the smoking jacket of the day, and not the customary tails to dinner. An American weekend guest at Sandringham had the Prince's Savile Row tailor make him a copy black Barathea double-breasted jacket, with satin lapels.

He wore this on his return to Tuxedo Park, New York. The heir of an American tobacco family wore a copy to the annual ball of the country club and caused much consternation. No one threw him out though because his father was club founder.

The jacket was an overnight sensation and soon became proper dress for formal evening wear. The present classic tuxedo has changed little from the Prince's jacket of 100 years ago.

STYLE

HAIRY TWEEDS AND TRAIL BLAZERS

In many a wardrobe hang city suits, dinner jackets and jeans and absolutely nothing in between. As one man put it, "I've got plenty of clothes but nothing to wear whenever I'm asked out for drinks or supper." So what to wear when a suit is too smart and casuals are too casual? The safest bet is to fall back on one of the old British standards – blazer and flannels or sports jacket and slacks, or a modern variation on the same theme, like a linen or cotton jacket with padded shoulders and deep pleated cotton slacks.

BLAZERS Blazers are not everyone's gin and tonic but a well cut blazer with the right kind of trimmings can be a very smart and adaptable garment. A 'good' traditional blazer is still quite likely to come in barathea, although there is a swing now to lighterweight wool. Double-breasted styles are both the most traditional and the most fashionable. The classic double-breasted blazer comes in barathea, while the fashion version will probably be in wool with a more up-to-date cut.

> "Familiar but not coarse, and elegant but not ostentatious."
> Samuel Johnson's definition of an English style. . .

Shirt cuffs are meant to show under a blazer as under a suit jacket and they are worn the same length. It is quite correct to wear a blazer with either plain coloured trousers, like flannels, or patterned slacks, like a discreet houndstooth check. The blazer and flannel combination is smart enough for a day in the office when there are no major meetings on the diary – a relaxed change from the usual suits.

Blazers come with two, three or even four buttons on vented cuffs. And buttons are the real giveaway when it comes to quality. Nothing makes a blazer look more bargain basement than pretend military buttons in embossed plastic. At the same time wearing authentic regimental buttons to which you are not entitled is really beyond the pale. A quality blazer will probably have gilt buttons or brass, although fashion blazers have started sporting fancy buttons like navy with gold rims, which makes them look more Italianate than country estate. Hackett, the elitist London tailors time-warped in the twenties and thirties, shun even hollow brass lacquered buttons. Says traditionalist managing director, Ashley Lloyd-Jennings, "Real brass buttons tarnish nicely and look good. Should you want them to shine you will, of course, clean them using your button stick." Just in case your home doesn't boast a button stick it is a brass plate with a slit up the middle, which you slip under your buttons to protect jacket material when you Brasso your buttons.

> The sports jacket is some 130 years old, having arrived in the 1850s as a suit jacket in sports club colours. Specifically for the rowing or rugger club it was not for wear in town. The young bloods later took to wearing it in town to the consternation of their elders.

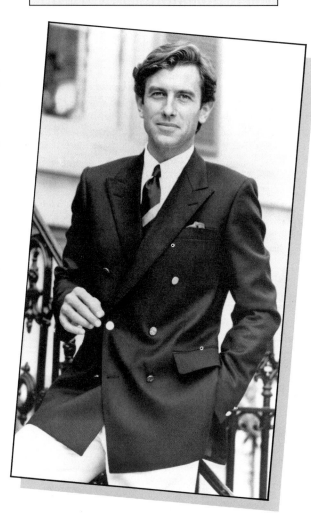

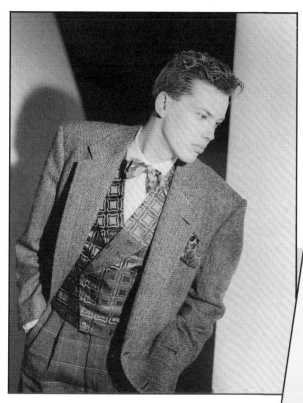

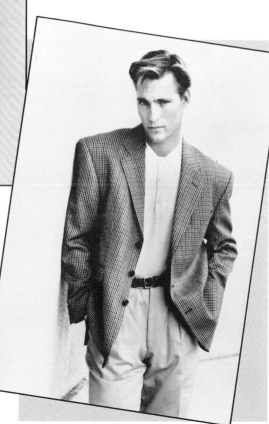

SPORTS JACKETS At Hackett, where sales staff are ex-public school and customers are city gents, country squires and army, sports jackets still come heavyweight and hairy. Not for them the move to softer, lightweight woollen cloth. Says Ashley Lloyd-Jennings, "Modern sports jackets are how the Italians consider Englishmen dress". But then Hackett are "very traditional and definitely not trendy or fashionable", to the extent of ignoring the fact that today's central heating hardly calls for the heavyweight tweeds of yesteryear.

Bespoke sports jackets at the top end of the price range come with real horn buttons, which are a natural mottled brown. The vents on sleeves have buttons which actually undo. Most off-the-peg jackets have buttons in either a toning horn effect or leather. Any kind of buttons are preferable to plastic masquerading as leather. The sleeves will be vented but buttons are unlikely to undo and on jackets at the bottom end of the price range the cuffs may not actually be split but have a sort of overlap cosmetic vent rather than a real one.

A hacking jacket style of sports jacket, with double vents at the back, is usually worn about an inch to an inch and a half longer, while the ordinary sports jacket, which comes without the nipped-in waist and skirt, is worn the same length as a suit jacket (the hem of which sits in your curled fingers with your hands straight by your sides).

People tend to wear these jackets half an inch longer in the sleeve and not show as much cuff, but there is no good reason for this. If you are going to wear an attractive shirt or sweater underneath you might as well flaunt it.

Patterned jackets should never be worn with patterned slacks – clashing checks are a sign of severe sartorial strife, not just a scuffle in the goalmouth at Sparta Prague.

A point worth remembering when buying a sports jacket is to see it more as a co-ordinate than as a separate. Give some thought to what you have got to wear with it. Trousers, shirts and sweaters should tone – pick out one of the colours in your jacket to match with your slacks. It is little use buying a Harris tweed in browns, creams and golds if most of your sweaters and slacks are grey and blue, and buying one pair of toning slacks which are 'dry clean only' will mean that you either leave the jacket in the wardrobe most of the time or go out looking like a mixed grill.

Most sports jackets are in wool, but they vary in weave and weight so decide what job you want yours to do. If it is to act mainly as a country casual for weekend walks go for a heavyweight; if it is to be a smart, casual indoor jacket try lightweight soft wool. But the great thing about this item of clothing is that whichever you go for it will adapt – a polo-neck sweater and corduroys will take your city jacket out of town while a white cotton shirt and club tie will take your country jacket in to supper.

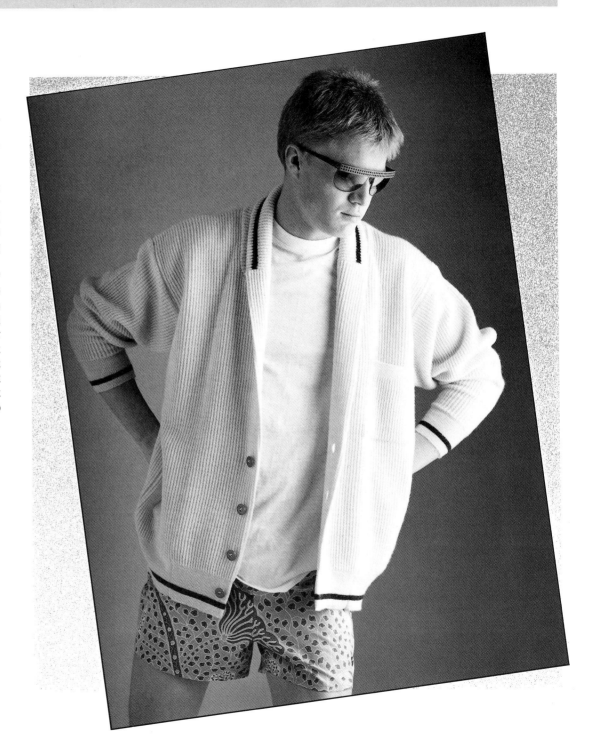

WHO'S WEARING THE TROUSERS

When it comes to trousers for leisure wear you will be spoilt for choice but make sure that you are not spoilt by it. Marks & Spencer, the ubiquitous British chainstore, alone have six ranges of off-duty trousers: denim, corduroy, pleated, luxury, classic and summer casuals. Have trousers will travel – the important question is where? Unless you have been invited to a barn dance denims no longer go out to dine and luxury slacks never leg it across the countryside unless you really want to look like wine bar man in the wolds. Luxury slacks will be all wool or a wool and polyester blend and they look best with blazer or sports jacket for smart casual wear. Cavalry twill, the country classic, will also team with a sports jacket, but they tend to look a bit old fashioned and country squire.

THREADS BARED It is when you hit the various blends that confusion can set in. Man-made fibre pick-'n'-mix trousers can have labels which are difficult to decipher.

Polyester is often labelled simply as polyester – a generic term – but you may find a brand name instead, especially Trevira, made by Hoechst. This is the main polyester used in the worsted style of trousers.

When you see 'worsted' on a label this is simply wool spun into a worsted. They take longer fibres and spin them finer, the name deriving from the birthplace of this technique in Norfolk.

You may see Lycra on a label. This is an elastane made by Du Pont, and used in very small percentages – something like two per cent – to give trousers stretch and shape retention.

Viscose, which you may know as rayon, used to be seen only at the cheapest end of the trouser range in a mix with polyester because viscose can be used as a cheaper substitute for worsted to stop the wind whistling through polyester. It is now often used as a fashion element as well because it can provide the sort of sheen which is currently popular.

When something is added to the mix it is often for designer reasons, not for wearability or washability. Hence linen may be added to cotton slacks or jackets because linen has a very natural, slightly 'slubby' look, which gives texture to the cloth.

If you see a permanent press label on slacks it means that the front crease should not wash out. A resin finish is put onto the fabric and then applying heat and pressure locks a memory into the cloth so that it remembers to retain the crease.

With 'best' trousers, as with suits, 100 per cent polyester fabric is seen as rather downmarket. If you do like 100 per cent polyester, however, remember that some polyester cloths can snag and go bobbly so discard slacks if they reach the *bouclé* stage. And try to select a softer fabric, not one that looks like an escaped McDonalds' uniform.

> *Eve Babitz said of President Richard Nixon, "I bet he wears a suit on the beach."*

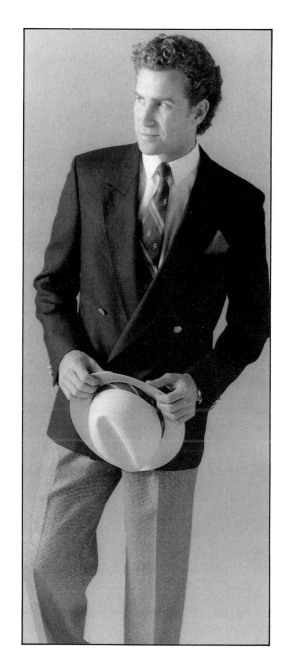

REBELS WITH A CAUSE – THE RIVETING FIGURES

"Blue jeans? They should be worn by farm girls milking cows," said Yves Saint-Laurent. The word denim is a contraction of '*serge de Nimes*', or serge of Nimes in southern France. The word jeans probably came from *Gênes*, French for Genoa. Both were stout twilled cotton fabrics used to make working clothes in Britain in the sixteen and seventeen hundreds. But in America they started using the word jeans to describe trousers made of the fabric. Then because they could hardly call them "jean jeans" the description denim jeans evolved, although strictly speaking both words mean the same thing.

Jeans, or denims, were restricted to the ranks of the workers or ranch hands until the 1950s. Then, glamorized by films like *Rebel Without A Cause*, blue jeans arrived on the urban scene. By the sixties British students had made blue jeans and T-shirts their uniform and in 1976 38 million pairs of jeans were sold in Britain and 170 million pairs were sold worldwide worth £1.6 billion, making Levi Strauss the world's biggest clothing manufacturer.

Latest figures show that sales in Britain have fallen to around 24 million pairs a year, which is still a lot of jeans. Most younger men still have at least one pair of jeans, but with casual wear smartening up jeans are beginning to return to their more rustic roots, unless they have particular street credibility like the riveting Levi 501s. No longer can you get away with wearing denim almost anywhere, and even at the very casual end of the trouser ranges corduroys and cotton slacks, both of which often come with front creases, have made considerable inroads.

Corduroy may well have got its name from *cord du roi* (cloth of kings) because the corded cotton had a pile like velvet. It was, however, just another farmworkers' fabric, which started life in the 18th century. Then intellectuals of the 1930s took to wearing corduroy trousers to show solidarity with the workers. These caught on and corduroy was also used for sportswear such as ski clothes and mountaineering breeches. They reached royal status

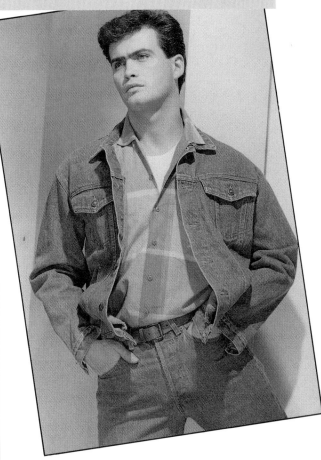

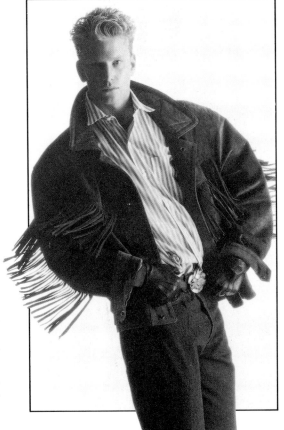

at last when the Prince of Wales wore them in the Austrian mountains. These days corduroys are worn heavyweight and chunky for the rugged, outdoors look, and soft and narrow for smarter wear. Alternatives are canvas trousers or lightweight cotton summer slacks.

Whichever casual trousers you opt for never kick about in them wearing your city shoes. This look is about as incongruous and comical as wearing swimming trunks with shoes and wooly socks. Casual trousers need casual shoes and leisure shirts – not the all-dressed-up variety.

Man-made fibres

A guide to terminology

SYNTHETICS
Oil based derivatives. Fibres based on products of the petrochemical industry. They include. . . .

POLYESTER: Most widely used man-made fibre, almost 20 per cent of all fibres used worldwide. Used alone or blended. In suits, trousers and in two-thirds of all shirts sold in the UK.

POLYAMIDE: Otherwise known as nylon. Sportswear or rainwear is often 100 per cent, socks are often blended with wool or cotton.

CELLULOSICS
Fibres deriving from wood pulp. They include. . .

VISCOSE: Otherwise known as rayon. The original man-made fibre, once termed artificial silk. Used alone or blended, often with polyester or cotton.

ACETATE and its refinement Triacetate: Ties and the silky linings in clothes are often made from these. Tricel, made by Courtaulds, is a recognizable brand name.

ACRYLIC: In the UK two-thirds of all knitwear is made of acrylic fibre. Courtelle, made by Courtaulds, is a well-known brand name and one of the earliest.

ELASTANE: Fibre used to give stretch and shape retention, Lycra is Du Pont's brand name. Used in stretch trousers, waistbands, cuffs, socks. Once called 'spandex'.

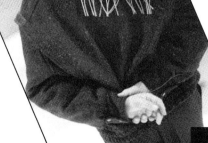

TATTERSALL OR TABLECLOTH

Country squire or country & western, check casual shirts can be colourful and comfortable. The upmarket Viyella variety come in a 55 per cent wool and 45 per cent cotton mix. But now Viyella, traditional mufti for retired colonels tending their vegetable gardens and seeing grandchildren through minor public schools, has added 100 per cent cotton twill to its range of classic 55 per cent wool/45 per cent cotton shirts.

Their designs are no longer all Tattersall check and houndstooth. One can hear the eyebrows rising in the shires as "vibrant bright colours" arrive to broaden Viyella's appeal. The classic Viyella will still be around for the few colonels left and they will still sell at about the same price as a ready-made Turnbull and Asser cotton shirt. The 100 per cent cotton shirts are staying upmarket in fabric quality, roomier fit, finish and price – about three times the cost of a chain store twilled cotton shirt. But then Viyella is seen as *la crème de la crème*, even if they are trying to spread it a little further. To ask if you can tell Viyella from the rest by its look is rather like applying the same test to a Jermyn Street shirt or Savile Row suit. It is for the upper crust rather than the crumbs and if you need to ask the price you probably can't afford it!

If you shop somewhat down the price range you can find attractive twilled cotton shirts in chain stores, or even at rock bottom prices in camping shops. The camping shop variety tend to be 'fun' shirts which look best with jeans. Take care with the checks though, bright colours are fine but the look to aim for is rugged outdoors, not truant gingham tablecloth.

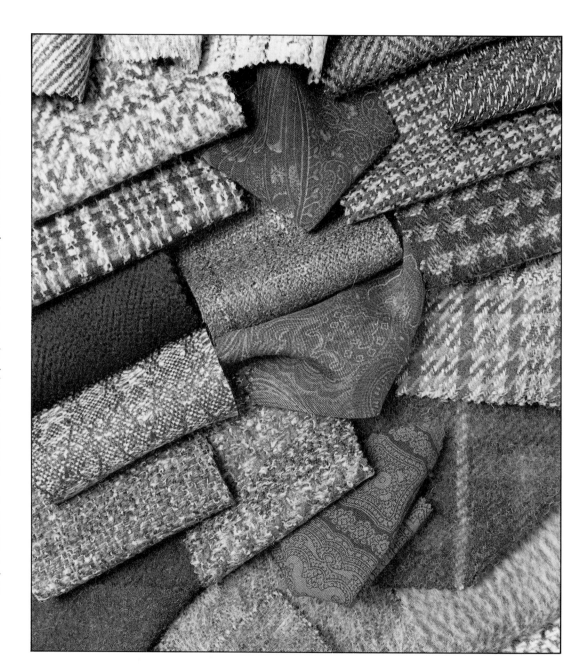

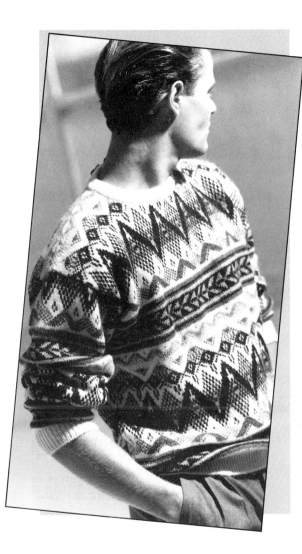

FEELING SHEEPISH

Once upon a time all woollies were just that. Now, since the birth and refinement of man-made fibres, two-thirds of all knitwear worn in the UK is made of acrylic fibre. And it is not just a question of cost, there is very little difference between the price of an all-wool or all-cotton sweater and one in an acrylic blend or 100 per cent acrylic.

Acrylic fibre is the most wool-like man-made fibre while being easier to look after than the real thing, but purists still do a ewe-turn at the sight of synthetic knitwear. They go for natural fibres, wool, wool and cotton blends, or cotton, and classic styles. Sabre, a company who concentrate on just such styles, specialize in polo shirts – knitted shirts with collar and placket and three or five buttons, crewnecks, roundnecked sweaters, and roll collars, polo-necks, so called to distinguish them from polo shirts, classic cardigans and knitted vests – the U name for waistcoats or sleeveless pullovers, and rather old hat.

Sabre knitwear, often with a salt and pepper tweedy look, is modelled by an aristocratic gent accompanied by a gun dog before a country manor or crackling log fire. This is 'quality' jersey land and it is reflected in the prices. Colours are all-important – their red is 'red enamel', their green 'viridian'. "Our colours are bright but sophisticated, we leave day-glo bright to the bottom end of the market", says the lady from Sabre.

The sort of sweater you can hear half a mile away does not usually have style unless it has a designer label.

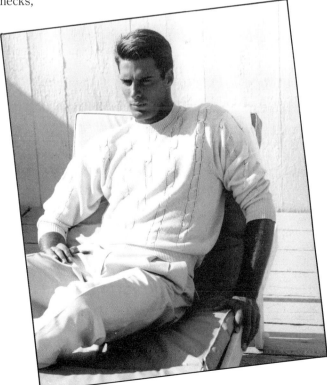

CLASS CHEAT If you want to dress upmarket but can't afford the cost you can buy a natural fibre sweater from a chainstore in a classic style for about two-thirds the price of a basic Sabre sweater. It won't look too different from one of its more aristocratic relations if you stick to safe colours.

If you are shopping cheap for an expensive look it takes a little *savoir-faire* though. Avoid lower caste logos, little chequered flags and the like (although some can be scratched off sweatshirts or unpicked if sewn on). It isn't just naff logos and lurid colours, however, shape and style matter too.

Street fashions may be baggy or boxy but the hons and upwards currently go for narrower, neater and not so sloppy heavyweight sweaters and looser fitting lightweights. Their cardigans are still comfortable but longer and leaner now, while their sweaters stop about mid-hip. The best way to cheat without getting caught is to identify the pricy garment you would like in an expensive shop and then toddle off downmarket to find the nearest copy. If in doubt about which logos or built in designer labels are acceptable don't fret, just reject the lot, because the days of wearing your labels on the outside have passed. Just one exception perhaps – the Lacoste crocodile.

Wearing a sweater under a suit might get you out of a spot if you are going somewhere without a clue about whether everyone will be formally or casually dressed. If you wear your suit with a shirt that's not too dressy and a classic sweater, you can always pocket your tie if it is a casual affair or park your sweater if it is formal.

ANORAKSIA NERVOSA

As with your city clothes the whole leisure package will come unstuck if the coat you cover it with lacks style. Petrol pump anoraks and nylon parkas with fake fur trim just won't do. A real arctic jacket that the huskies wouldn't howl at is a different matter.

Casual jackets come in a multitude of types and with a multitude of titles – ski jackets, blousons, parkas, anoraks, wadded or padded. Nobody agrees on the terminology – one store's anorak is another store's parka. To be acceptable it simply has to look stylish and not as if you picked it up on a petrol station forecourt with the four-star or in a local cheapo camping shop.

Colours have arrived in a big way and some combinations look very classy. The 'all things bright and beautiful' style of jacket is for true casual wear, fine on a touchline but not for arriving at the boss's drinks party.

For Sloanes the Barbour is *de rigueur*. This dark olive green oilcloth with the cord collar, once confined to rural weatherproofing, has been taken up in a big way by the 'Fulham Farmers' and it is easy to see why. A Barbour is wind and waterproof, not merely shower resistant, it doesn't date and is one of those garments which improves with age. If the rest of your casual clothes wouldn't look too out of place at a point-to-point a Barbour would cover it. Even though the real thing is not cheap it will outlast a fashion anorak.

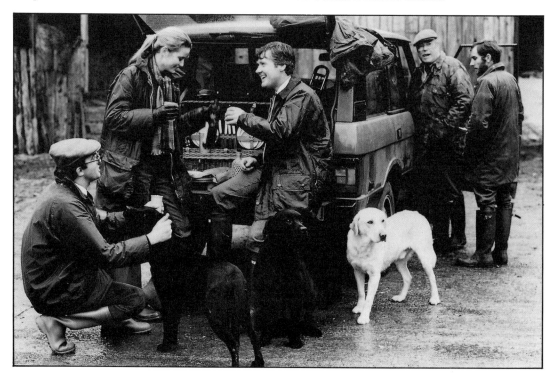

NICE LEGS, SHAME ABOUT THE RACE

If you run for sport or fun and not just to catch a bus beware, the sportswear manufacturers may have designs on your legs in no time.

"Tights," says the gentleman from Nike (pronounced Nikey if you want to sound like a real sportsman), "are very popular now. An increasing number of sports stars are wearing them and if you go down to a local running track one night you will see lots of men training in tights." True enough there they are, pounding down the tartan in something very akin to their girlfriends' aerobics outfits. . . .

If you can't quite take to tights but still want to look like a real athlete when you go out for a run forget the straight-legged fashion track suit or the fleecy lined jogging bottoms: the good old functional tapered leg with zips up the sides are back. And although the extrovert can still buy dramatic colour combinations, maniac dogs are less offended by runners in traditional sports colours like navy, black, royal, red and grey. It matters not whether your track suit comes from the Nike, Adidas, Puma end of the range or the Lacoste, Head, Ellesse pricy end if you are good, but if your running style is a bit of a joke don't dress it up, dress it down.

Singlets should be the real thing because although based on the vest shape there are important differences like lightweight materials and the fact that they are cut very high on the shoulders to stop them slipping down. Nothing looks less macho than a man who has to keep hitching up his shoulder straps. Shorts should be brief with a split leg to allow movement and built in liner. And for the British winter there is nothing to beat thermal running underwear.

In wet weather the ultimate weatherproofing is an expensive Gore-Tex suit in three-ply fabric with a Gore-Tex membrane in the middle, meant to let moisture out but not to let rain in. These cost about three times the price of a decent track suit and most runners, Steve Cram included, go for cheap nylon suits, which keep them relatively warm and dry.

When it's anyone for tennis or squash the traditional look has resurfaced here too. It is more well-bred than brat now – the white shirt with green collar stripe, cool classic rather than cluttered McEnroe look. The Fred Perry range is one of the most popular because it looks good and isn't wildly expensive.

Never play squash in running shoes unless you want injuries, because the built-up sole of a running shoe is not designed for the game, and go for a proper track suit for cover-up or warm-up wear. Jogging suits are more casual clothes, for the man who wants to look sporty rather than the sportsman. Jason Jogging Suit (his gear probably comes bestriped from a chainstore and his running shoes are spotless) probably runs no further than from his badly parked Golf convertible to the kerb.

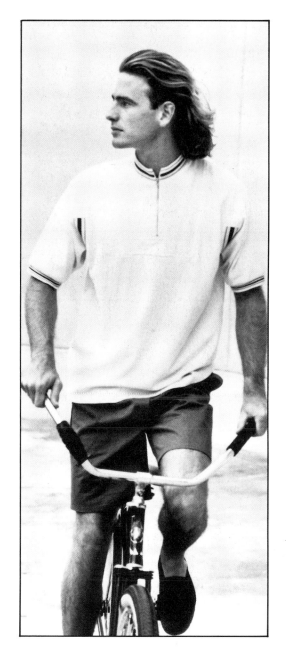

Little things mean a lot

In the city where any colour suit will do as long as it is grey the only way to add sparkle to your appearance is with the little things in life. Ties, shoes, socks, pocket handkerchiefs are not merely part of a uniform or functional items, they are often the only means of hauling your image out of the humdrum and putting it on the map.

If you are going out to dinner or you have been invited away for the weekend it is often the bare accessories that let you down – the plastic belt, the tacky matching tie and handkerchief set, the city shoes to tread the woodlands. Frequently the carefully-chosen suit or elegant casuals are simply reduced to the rubbish heap by cheap shoes or bad taste ties. An aspiring Smarty Artie becomes merely Boring Boris when his completed outfit is so drab that finding his socks and tie is like looking for a grey cat on a foggy day.

> *Nowadays more than six hundred million people wear ties every day.*

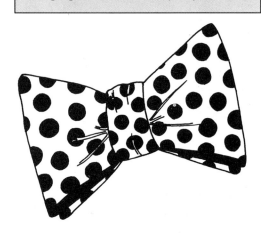

THE TIE THAT CAME IN FROM THE COLD

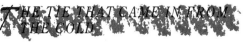

It is generally thought that today's necktie began life as a sort of scarf. Until recently historians believed that the Roman legionaries started it all. The earliest scarves featured on the 40 metre high Column of Trajan, erected in Rome in 113 AD after the emperor Trajan's soldiers vanquished the Dacian barbarians. Today you can still see the imperial legionaries wearing lengths of material around their necks, some tucked into their armour and others worn knotted like cowboy neckerchiefs.

But then in 1974 Chinese peasants digging a well discovered part of the tomb of Shih Huang Ti, the tyrannical first emperor of China, who forced millions of men to build the Great Wall.

Buried along with him in 210 BC was an army of no less than seven thousand five hundred terracotta soldiers, each wearing a scarf.

It seems that the scarves of the Romans and Chinese were only worn by the military, most likely to stop armour chafing or to keep the elements at bay. When the cravat, the nearest relation to the modern tie, surfaced it also appeared in a military context. Louis XIII hired a regiment of Central European Croat mercenaries during the Thirty Years War. This cavalry regiment, the '*Cravate Royale*', wore their wide collars tied in a knot, a custom which became adopted and adapted in European dress.

But whereas the ancient scarves had a purpose, our ties are purely decorative. By 1828 all the English dandies were studying 22 ways of tying a cravat in the best-seller, *The Art of Tying a Cravat* by H. Le Blanc. It now seems likely that this was a pseudonym of Honoré de Balzac, who it is thought wrote it, including a list of tradesmen, to pacify and buy off tie maker and shirt maker creditors. At this time a man-about-town wore at least 30 different necker-chiefs in a single week.

Towards the second half of the nineteenth century the narrower necktie appeared as collars shrank in size and became less stiff and less strangulation tight. Since then they have been an essential part of Western dress.

But why has the tie survived when it is really the only item of men's clothing that serves no useful purpose? Some psychologists link its popularity with the suggestion that it is a phallic symbol. But the tie's abiding appeal lies more in the fact that it is the one article of clothing with which men can really make a statement and with which they can say something different every day.

> "Why do you always wear a tie?"
> "Because I play a lot of strip poker –
> badly. . ."   Anon.

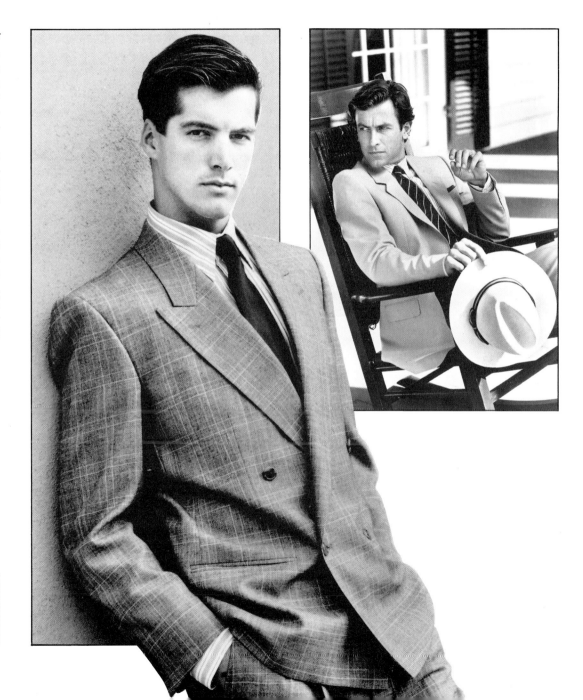

> *One of the biggest collections of regimental, club and company ties is on display at the Bear Inn, Alfred Street, Oxford. Here more than 7000 tie pieces are displayed. Drinkers allowing the landlord to cut the end of a tie missing from the collection usually get a pint on the house.*

> *"When he buys his ties he has to ask if gin will make them run."*
> F. Scott Fitzgerald

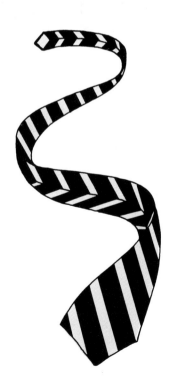

TAKING SILK Some men have one tie in their wardrobe and some have twenty – anybody who really cares about his appearance will have a good selection. It is little use, though, having fifteen or twenty ties if most are unwearable either because they have gone out of style or because they are too bedraggled or grubby. Weeding is called for if you are not always to be seen in the same couple of ties because all the others can't be worn but convince you that you have got plenty.

If you are pruning your stock of neckwear consider a rethink of material if you have always bought polyester. Silk ties are no longer the prerogative of the well-to-do, and buying polyester because it is washable is a bit pointless if you seldom wash your ties anyway.

If you stand in front of a display of ties in a store after some preliminary look-and-feel testing you will probably be able to recognize the ones in silk. They will need more looking after than polyester, but if you are going to upgrade the fabric of your suit then try a silk tie as well.

It's now possible to buy silk ties at prices you may well have paid in the past for polyester as more and more chainstores take to silk. Will Hobhouse, managing director of the Tie Rack, a chain of shops specializing in ties, says that although 70 per cent of all ties sold in the UK are polyester, his company sells 70 per cent in silk and men are gradually becoming more aware when it comes to fashion and fabrics. Once you have persuaded yourself to pay just a little extra for silk you might decide it is worth travelling even further upmarket, going for a quality tie in a better, heavier silk.

KNOTTY PROBLEMS Most ties measure 56 and a half inches end to end and when tied the blade is supposed to rest just at the top of your waistband. If you are average height you will probably need to start with the broad end about

ten inches longer than the narrow end before you begin tying the knot. This will need adjusting according to the type of knot but when adjusted you should still have enough at the narrow end to slot through the loop on the back of the blade designed to hold it in place.

Fat Windsor knots should not be used with button-down collars and tweeds and knitted ties belong with sports jackets not city suits. Never wear the label on the outside, a signed tie only labels your insecurity. Knots should never be pulled too tight or undone with a tug: undo the knot properly unless you want to break the fibres and pucker the tie.

Don't choose a tie the same colour as your suit unless it's an exact match, find one that complements it. Some shops keep suit swatches for this purpose. Don't simply drop your tie over the back of a chair at the end of a hard day. If you want it fit to wear again hang it up properly on a proper rail in your wardrobe or on a tie rack. And never put your tie on half way through a snatched breakfast: fingers fresh from buttering toast will only add another print to the pattern.

BOW BRUMMELLS It is difficult to know why grown men insist on wearing hook-on bow ties particularly if they often wear this style of neckwear. The bow tied is only the same as the one tied to do up shoelaces and if an eight-year-old can learn to tie a school tie any man ought to be able to cope with a bow tie and not resort to buying them ready tied.

It may seem that with so many different designs on today's ties selecting one from among them all is an impossible task. But the vast array fall into less than ten basic categories. . .

DESIGNS ON YOU

PERFECTLY PLAIN
A tie of one solid colour, either eye-catching or conservative. Every wardrobe should have one as they can be worn with any combination of suit and shirt pattern.

TOTALLY DOTTY
From micro-dots to polka-dots. Elegant and versatile, these too will team with any shirt and suit. The smaller the dot the more formal the tie.

REGIMENT OF STRIPES
Based on regimental or old school ties these come in many combinations of colours and striped in any combination of widths. An old rule is never to wear suit, shirt and tie in three different patterns but rules were made to be broken, especially if done with flair.

PAISLEY PERSUASION
Useful ties to mix and match because they combine several colours. The brighter coloured ones are traditionally sporty, the darker, more subdued version dressy.

CLUB TYPES
These are ties with regularly spaced club-type motifs, like heraldic shields or sporting motifs. Genuine club ties should only be worn by those entitled to them.

REGULAR GUY
Sometimes called foulard, *these feature a series of regularly spaced small designs like flower shapes, diamonds or circles, or a combination of them, on a plain background. As with paisley the subdued version is the more formal.*

GEOMETRY SET
Any geometric pattern running across a tie from intricate zig-zags to large diamond patterns. Generally speaking the larger the pattern the more casual the tie.

HIGHLAND FLING
Plaids and checks have traditionally been regarded as casual ties, the heavier woollen version often being worn with tweed jackets. There is no reason why sleeker versions shouldn't be worn with a suit though.

FLOWER POWER
Some rather lovely ties are made in open floral Liberty-style designs. Attractive with the right outfit but too pretty for macho man or sober sides.

Plain

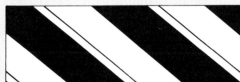

Dots

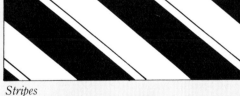

Stripes

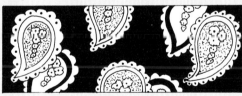

Paisley

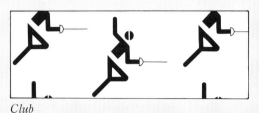

Club

Foulard

Geometric

Plaid

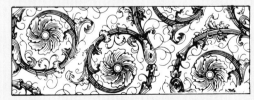

Floral

S
T
Y
L
E

*T*YING THE KNOT

There are three standard types of knot – the basic Four-In-Hand, the Half-Windsor and the Windsor.

Four-in-Hand   *When heavy fabric would give an overly large Windsor knot and for button-down and longer close-point collars.*

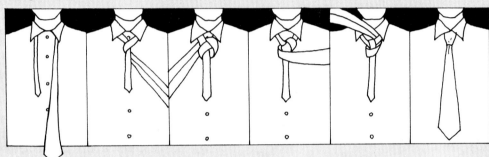

Half-Windsor   *More triangular. Fits well with standard or widish spread collars. Better than a Windsor for wide or thick ties.*

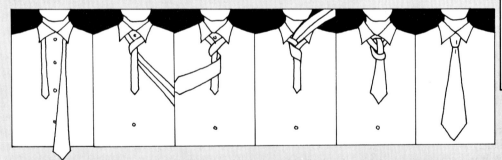

Windsor   *Stylish with a sleek tie and a wide spaced collar.*

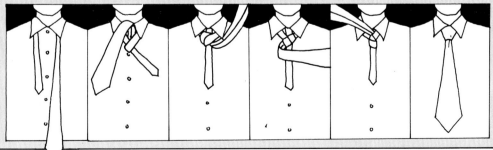

Bow Tie   *Normal for formal, a bit daring for everyday.*

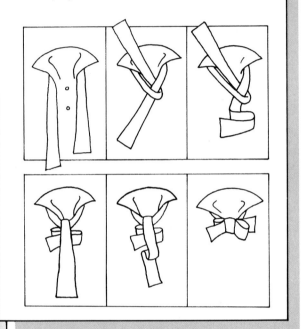

If you are considering wearing a bow tie every day take care: while acceptable in more flamboyant fields, the more sombre professional boss would probably prefer you staid in an ordinary tie.

> *"A well-tied tie is the first serious step in life."*   Oscar Wilde

FRENCH STYLE In the stock market where men watch their appearance as closely as clients' cash, the moneyed, sophisticated look is the thing. Any old silk tie won't do, Hermès ties (pronounced 'Ermez', français-style) are *de rigueur*. Said one young investment banker, "I'd rather not wear a tie if it is not a Hermès tie, although perhaps a Jaeger one would do." Hermès wisely have a branch at the Royal Exchange as well as in New Bond Street. Twice the price of a silk tie from Turnbull & Asser, their ties, which are made in Lyons, are so expensive, say Hermès, because of the original designs, perfect cut and quality of the silk. "Only two ties are made out of a metre of silk, the only join is down the back, they are all hand finished and lined with good quality silk. They are usually worn by people like bankers, lawyers, certain politicians and captains of industry. Oh, and royalty, of course," said the lady from "Ermez". . . .

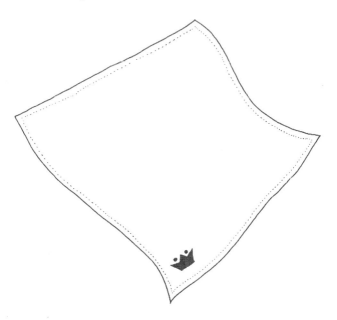

HANKY-PANKY

If the Englishman wears a handkerchief in his breast pocket he usually opts for one that matches his tie exactly – *ergo* he is incapable of making two sound decisions at the same time. On the continent they manage it and even in America, but as with his co-ordinating shirt and tie set Mr Lethargic of Luton takes the easy way out. "The level of sophistication here is still really rather low," reflected one necktie manufacturer sadly, "although men are gradually becoming weaned onto wearing different ties and handkerchiefs." If you want to show some style don't duplicate your tie, select a colour from it and repeat that in your pocket handkerchief.

Some style guides give as many as eight or ten ways to fold your "pocket square" – forget them. Reject the mountain peaks, especially those attached to bits of card or, worse still, credit card holders or notebooks (can you imagine anyone lifting out their hanky only to reveal a scrap of cloth atop a "useful" notepad!). Shun too the neatly folded rectangle which looks, as someone acidly put it, as if you have forgotten to post your pools coupon.

The stylish way to do it is to make your handkerchief look as though it has simply been casually pocketed. To do this lay it down flat, pick it up by the centre, poke the points down into the pocket and leave the centre patch protruding about half an inch – *voila*! the gentleman's handkerchief.

> *The handkerchief is 600 years old and Richard II is credited with its invention, having been above the normal custom of blowing the nose on a sleeve or onto the floor.*

UNDERCOVER AGENTS

Away with your Y-fronts if you don't want to look ridiculous to women. Knickerbox, the men's and women's undies chain, discovered in a survey that some 24 per cent of the ladies think men look ridiculous in their underwear, particularly in Y-fronts. About 62 per cent think that boxer shorts and briefs are sexy though – a fact that Knickerbox probably realized when the Levi jeans advertisement featuring a chap stripping down to his shorts to wash his jeans at the launderette sent sales of boxer shorts soaring.

It is usually the maxi and micro underpants that raise a laugh and deflate male ego. The posing pouch approach is out for the heterosexual male who doesn't want his girlfriend in fits of giggles, and trendy grans often try to persuade their menfolk out of the bell-tent bloomers of yesteryear and into something more appealing.

Knickerbox, who set up shop expecting sales of 80 per cent women's undies and 20 per cent men's found that selling soon almost reached 50 per cent for each, although more than half the men's pants are bought for them by women. Among the best-sellers are pure silk boxer shorts and briefs, "We sell them in bright blue, red, black and white and have introduced pale colours like pink and cream. Men come in and buy six pairs at a time, which has amazed us. But they are extremely sexy and feel wonderful," says Janie Godber, Knickerbox's design director.

Briefs still outsell shorts, selling at least double the numbers. But it's likely that this will change as there is a tremendous call now for boxer shorts for boys of 11 upwards.

BIT PARTS AND NIGHTS ERRANT Underpants sizes are based on waist measurements. Small are usually 28–30, medium 32–34 and large 36–38, and sometimes they come in extra large too. Men don't always realize the basis of sizing though. According to Knickerbox they fight shy of asking for 'small' undies. "Girls will buy small pants for their men but the men themselves won't," said Janie Godber. "We usually make a point of asking for their waist size so there is no misunderstanding."

Turnbull & Asser sell boxer shorts which match their shirts and sales have recently increased tenfold. They sell pyjamas and dressing gowns in their shirting materials too. But men often wear their boxer shorts to bed, if they wear anything at all. Sales of pyjamas only amount to 0.2 pairs per man per year and younger men tend never to buy any. One famous chainstore has found selling pyjamas an increasingly uphill struggle and introduced double packs of trousers only. Birthday suit bedwear is simply a return to tradition. Everyone slept in the nude until the nightshirt appeared on the scene in the sixteenth century – although they did often wear nightcaps. . . .

> *"His socks compelled one's attention without losing one's respect."*
> Saki

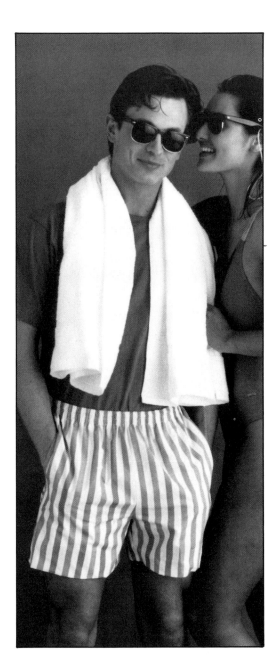

SOCKING IT TO THEM

If you can add a splash of colour to your sober city suit with the right tie there is no reason why you can't add a dash more with your socks. Patterned ankles, once thought too racy for the wage rats, are now becoming an acceptable way to display individual style and a sense of the slightly humorous. As with bow ties the really lively ones won't go down too well in more sober circles but you won't put your foot in it with more subtle patterns.

These days Argyles are everywhere, in multi-coloured gaiety or muted mix and match. Men have also realized that too heavy a dose of man-made fibres can make feet smell less than lovely. Natural fibres and wool-rich and cotton-rich blends are less likely to walk down the stairs on their own at the end of a busy day.

A real bonus for men with naturally noxious feet is a sock called the Burlington Argyle, a one-size sock in 75 per cent acrylic 25 per cent nylon with its own built in deodorant called 'Bioguard', which actually works and prevents fungus problems too. These soft, fluffy socks come in a multitude of colours from gentlemanly grey to pinks and purples. They are not cheap, nor are they long-wearing, but they do solve the foul feet problem and they do look good. The Sock Shop and major department stores sell them, and one upmarket shop said that though they used to keep both traditional woollen gents' socks and Burlingtons, they had phased the woollens out because everyone wanted the Argyles.

The Sock Shop chain say that men are switching from traditional plain black and plain grey in favour of brighter colours. Favourite fabrics are acrylic and cotton mix, 100 per cent cotton, 100 per cent wool in winter, silk, silk lookalikes and particularly the Burlington range.

BELTING UP

A belt may keep your trousers up but let your image down. No item of clothing is there merely to perform a function, if it is on display it should look right too. A formal suit calls for a smart belt, not one that came free with your last pair of corduroys.

If you have a couple of suits and several pairs of casual trousers you should have a selection of belts too. One belt won't look right with everything. The ideal belt for the city suit comes in plain leather and has an elegant, not an overstated buckle (forget the Gucci insignia), it should tone with the rest of your outfit and not look like an outsider.

With casual trousers and jeans fabric belts in plain or striped toning colours are fine as is a less classic leather belt. Buckles too can be less restrained, although cowboy memorabilia like six-guns and galloping horses are best left to the kids and country & western fans. Generally, fabric, leather-trimmed fabric or leather belts all serve a purpose, but plastic belts always look tacky unless they work on a gimmicky level.

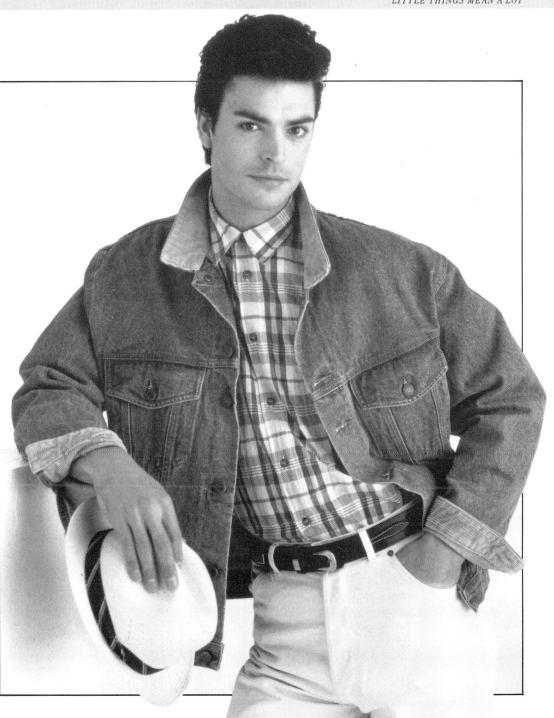

ANOTHER MAN'S SHOES

Shoes have always been one of the most functional items of clothing since early man made primitive sandals out of grass, strips of hide or pieces of wood to protect his feet. They were invented of necessity and developed according to the needs of those wearing them.

The Egyptians, one of the first civilized people to make footwear, bound pads of leather or papyrus to their feet with two straps and sometimes turned the front up to protect their toes. The Romans took the sandal a step further with a series of straps knotted on top of the foot. Eskimos and Indians, exposed to extreme cold, tied bags of grass around their feet, which developed into moccasins.

Shoes are heavily symbolic too. Dying with your shoes on originally meant going to the gallows, and 'waiting for dead men's shoes' came from an old custom of beneficiaries of an inheritance removing the dead person's shoes. There used to be a custom too of adopted sons donning their new father's shoes – stepping into their shoes, in fact.

> *"A shoe too large trips you up."*
> *A Latin proverb roughly equivalent to the present day saying,*
> *"Getting too big for your boots."*

But while shoes have always served a purpose they have been subject to the whims of fashion too. Sometimes they have been as much of a hazard as a protection. When those incredibly long-toed shoes were all the rage in the fourteenth century the French aristocrats even went to war in them. In the Battle of Poitiers in 1356 they had to advance on a narrow front which meant getting off their horses and walking, impossible in their shoes. They had to cut the ends off their shoes before they could advance, lost the battle and saw their king taken prisoner.

High heels on men's shoes arrived in the 1600s with two-inch heels. They were revived by young London beaux in the late 1700s and again with the high heeled boots of the 1960s.

AT A PINCH Whatever style of shoes you choose it is important to ensure that they are a comfortable fit when you buy them. Shopping towards the end of the day when your feet have swollen will stop you buying footwear that will feel too tight later. Never buy shoes without trying them on properly – different makers' sizes differ in both width and length so don't just assume that because they are your usual size they will fit.

Everyone has odd feet so buy for the bigger one, usually the right foot, and ignore salesmen's patter about "breaking them in", if they are too tight don't buy them. Allow half an inch between the tips of your toes and your shoes and make sure they are not tight over the instep. If you can lace a lace-up so that the two edges meet, try a narrower one. And try to buy the shoes you wear for work with leather uppers – they will adapt to the shape of your feet and allow them to breathe.

> *It used to be said that to put the left shoe on before the right or shoes on the wrong feet was unlucky, after Augustus Caesar got his shoes in a muddle and was almost assassinated on the same day.*

> *"Calceos mutare" – A Roman saying, literally to change one's shoes, meaning to become a senator, the highest social rank.*

> *Shoes got involved in weddings too, with the custom of throwing old shoes or tying them to the wedding car, thought to be a relic of ancient laws of exchange in which a bride's parents gave up all rights over her.*

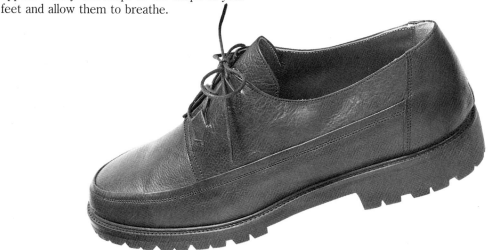

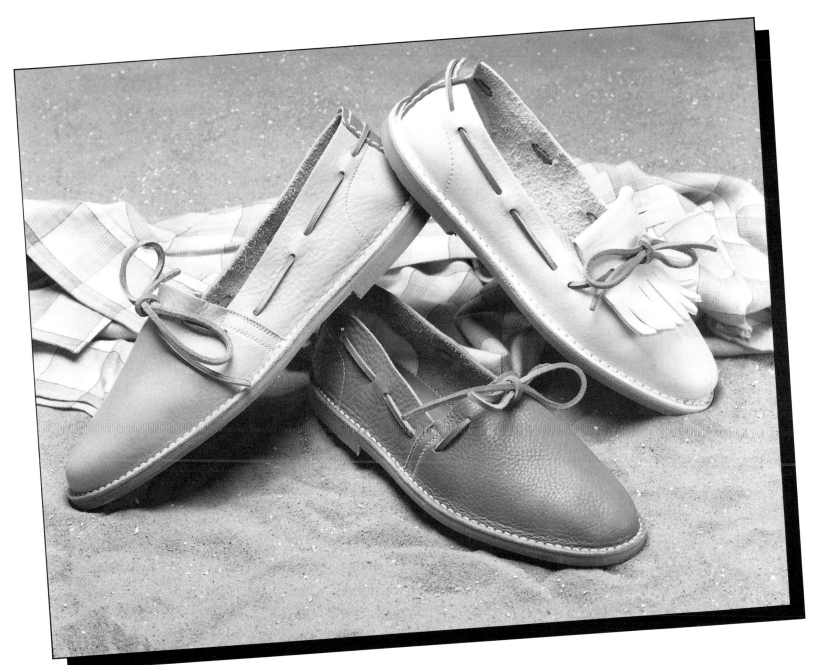

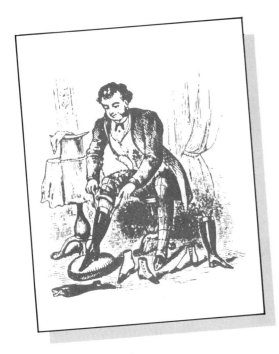

STEPPING INTO THE RIGHT SHOES In ancient Rome the type of shoes you wore depended on your rank and status and nothing much has changed. Today a man can still be categorized by his shoes whether they are mass-produced, cheap import shoes with man-made uppers and stuck-on man-made soles, which will soon wear out or fall apart and be dumped in the bin, or a pair of shoes in the finest leather, meticulously handcrafted, which, if looked after, could last more than twenty years.

A man who has found his feet and the wherewithal to cover them with style often opts for "Church's Famous English Shoes" and 115 years of British craftsmanship. A Church's shoe is made by a series of some 250 separate operations and bears a title worthy of its pedigree – Henley, Balmoral, Mayfair, Brigade. Their slippers have names too – like Hercules II, Perseus IV, Hermes II; you can almost hear a Church's gent calling his slippers to fetch the dog.

FEET OF CLAY According to the British Shoe Corporation black is still the most popular colour for men's shoes, followed by grey and navy blue. But men are becoming more daring, taking on board boat shoes and accepting colour trims in their stride.

Classic Oxfords, with plain toe caps or brogues, have long been the standard uniform for professional men. Decorative perforation on shoes actually started out serving a useful purpose. In Ireland and Scotland people's *brogs* (shoes) kept getting waterlogged on marshy land and someone hit on the idea of punching holes in them to let the water out and some ventilation in. At the end of the 19th century shoemakers began copying the pattern onto more modern shoes.

Shoe styling is moving away from very tapered toe caps in favour of a slightly heavier look with tyre-tread soles, and a smarter version of a traditional loafer can now be worn with a business suit.

In fact, even as Church's Famous English shoes head across the Atlantic bound for America, so traditional American loafers pass them *en route* to fashionable up market shops in London's Covent Garden and Kings Road. Many of the American shoes have almost reached the price of Church's by the time they get here. Tassel loafers, with the knotted lace and tassels on the front, and penny loafers, the bar with a money box slot originally for holding a dime, luxuriate in names like Sebago Docksiders and Bass Wee-juns and they have a lot of street credibility among the well-heeled young.

Well Heeled?

Figures supplied by The British Shoe Corporation Limited

MENS SHOES PURCHASED

Age Group	12–24	25–34	35–44	45–54	55+
Average pairs per year	5.7	4.3	3.3	2.8	1.9

MONEY SPENT

Age Group		12–24	25–34	35–44	45–54	55+
Average amount spent yearly	£	93.59	76.26	58.25	48.25	28.26

Taking off your shoes is a mark of respect in many countries and often shoes are left at the door of a place of worship.

FAST MOVER OR STICK-IN-THE-MUD Boat shoe casuals and jazzy plimsolls or deck shoes are at the fun end of leisure footwear and a lot of running shoes are sold to people who want to walk, not run too. If you are looking for trainers to lounge in or to do a little jogging the cheapest end of the Hi-Tech and Reebok ranges are as good as the more expensive shoes. But if you want to do more serious running Nike air soles are worth investing in: they are extremely comfortable to wear and give a good run for your money.

Heading off the beaten track and you will need wellies. Even down among the Wellington boots, originally leather and named after the Duke of Wellington, there's a style divide. You can opt for black workman wellingtons or sea green gentleman farmer's boots. Uniroyal's 'Hunter' style green wellies have even crossed the Atlantic, to a warm welcome from Americans used to stiff, black rubber 'barn boots'. "Kind of stylish, kind of daring," enthused an American magazine. Meanwhile, Barbour now have their own wellies too, in a darker green and blue, also made by Uniroyal but to Barbour's specifications.

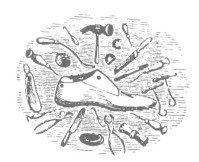

Singing in the Rain

Up until the early 1800s gentlemen carried canes not umbrellas, which when they first appeared were thought far from manly. Then umbrellas were taken up by the dandies and the army. During action at Bayonne in 1813 guards officers put up their umbrellas in the rain, which appalled the Duke of Wellington, who sent instructions that the Guards could carry umbrellas on parade but not under fire.

Gentlemen never carry umbrellas in the country unless to keep the womenfolk dry at a garden fête or some dressy event. And if you want to look good carrying an umbrella, the only one allowable is a gentleman's rolled umbrella in black. Forget all those strange truncated brollies that amputate fingertips in their telescopic action – the blood looks bad on a shirt front and men look silly carrying them anyway.

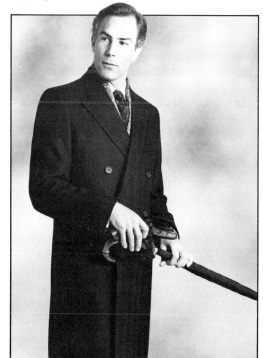

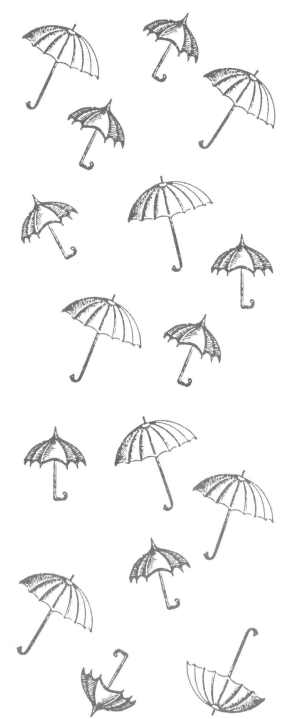

How green was my valet

Unless you have in your employ a gentleman's gentleman the chances are that you will have to do some valeting yourself now that the womenfolk have rebelled.

Don't know how? Here are some useful hints to help you iron out the wrinkles.

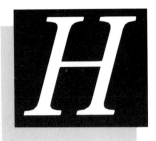

PRESSED TO IMPRESS

The professional's way to press a pair of trousers. Courtesy of Josie Burles, who presses and hand finishes suits at Moss Bros Covent Garden headquarters and also "looks after the directors' clothes".

1. "Take a damp cloth at least 18 inches square. A piece of old cotton sheet or an old tea cloth will do, something soft and well-used with no starch or finish in it, as stiff cotton won't hold the water and you will get a gloss on the material.

2. Have the iron setting on hot but make sure you do not touch the trousers with it as you will get an almost unmovable shine. Press the waist band first. Then pull the pockets inside out and iron those. Keep the pockets out and press the trousers, working from the top of the fly down to the bottom of the leg. If you keep your two seams together you will have a straight crease.

3. Do not keep your iron on the material until it is dry as this will produce a gloss, pick it up when the pressing cloth is still slightly damp.

4. Then you have to use a piece of wood, a small, smooth piece with no rough edges. Bang it down onto the material to absorb all the moisture and flatten the seams.

5. If you don't use a piece of wood but a thick piece of dry cloth and your iron again, do this very lightly and be careful not to create a shine. It is no good just hanging the trousers up in a warm place while still damp because what you are trying to do is to press the crease in while absorbing the moisture. Simply hanging them means they won't hold the crease."

If you doubt your expertise with an iron you could invest the price of one decent suit in buying a trouser press. The best-known are made by Corby of Windsor.

Often called simply Corby's they are to be found lurking in many hotel bedrooms, in lieu of the old-fashioned valet service. These gadgets, which come either free-standing or for mounting on the wall, resemble an upright convector heater, eating a pair of trousers. They are guaranteed for two years, safe on man-made fibres or the softest pure wool, and give a "shape-up" in 15 minutes and a "full press" in 30 minutes.

Alternatively a high street dry cleaners can usually dry clean your suit in two hours or press it while you wait. One dry cleaner reports: "Pressing will take five to ten minutes. We have had desperate customers coming in and waiting in the loo while we pressed the suit they came in wearing."

RUNNING REPAIRS

Reputable dry cleaners will also often take on all types of repairs and alterations, shortening or lengthening sleeves, replacing trouser zips and waist fastenings, taking trousers in. They will also send damaged garments away for invisible mending. Such calamities as cigarette burns can be dealt with by this process, which involves delicate work under a magnifying glass, taking a piece of material from inside the garment and weaving it back in using threads out of the material.

GETTING THE BRUSH-OFF

Brush suits, jackets and trousers regularly with a fine, firm-bristled brush. If a garment needs a tidy-up when there is no clothes brush handy, sticky tape wrapped around the closed fingers of one hand will remove dust and fluff. . . .

JUST HANGING AROUND

Empty your pockets before putting clothes away and do not use a dry cleaner's wire hanger for your suit, jacket or slacks. Jackets should be hung on substantial hangers wide enough to support the shoulders and trousers on the rung of a decent hanger to avoid creasing and wrinkles. Don't pack clothes into the wardrobe so tightly that they don't have room to breathe. . . .

DRY BARBOURS NEED FEEDING

Barbour jackets and lookalikes have to be treated with proper waterproof dressing when they dry out. Barbour's own 'Thornproof Dressing' should be available from shops selling the jackets. Apply to the whole garment or to patches prone to drying out, like elbows. . . .

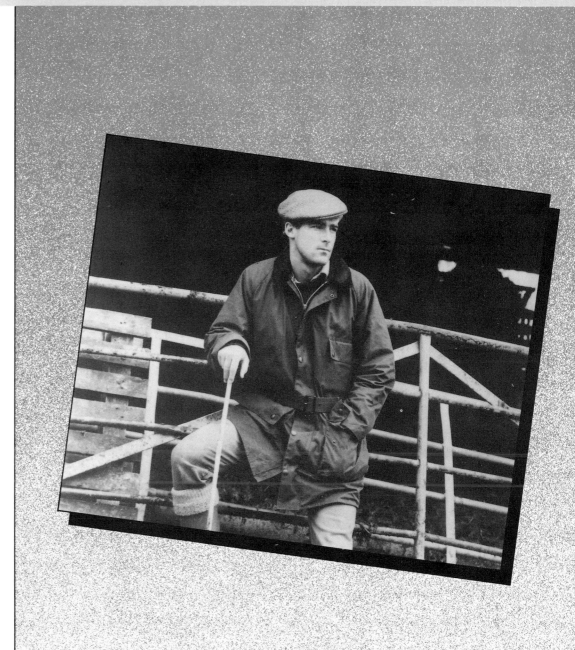

Putting on the Ritz

*The right way to iron and fold a shirt,
courtesy of David, valet at the Ritz*

1. Set the iron on a suitable setting.
2. First iron the yoke, then the cuffs, then the sleeves, then the collar, followed by the left front, and the back, finishing with the right front so that you finish with the shirt facing you.
3. Button the shirt all the way down.
4. Turn it face down and smooth it out.
5. Lift one side and fold it one third towards the centre of the back, take the sleeve and lay it neatly over the fold.
6. Lift the other side and fold that one third towards the centre, take the other sleeve and lay that neatly over the fold.
7. Fold the bottom of the shirt, including the tail, up. The fold should come at a line across the shirt, exactly below the cuffs.
8. Fold the whole thing in half.
9. Turn it over and you should have a shirt which looks as if it has just returned from the laundry.

SPRAYING AWAY WITH A SMOOTH IRON Shirts, particularly cotton ones, are easier to iron when damp and not absolutely dry. If your shirt is completely dry use a plant spray mister (available in hardware stores) to dampen it as you iron.

You may prefer spray starch but beware the sort that leaves your shirt with a flaky dandruff after ironing. Some really keen types put their shirt in a polythene bag and leave it in the salad crisper section of the refrigerator for a couple of hours because using a hot iron on the cold shirt gives a really crisp finish. . .

> *"He's a man out there in the blue, riding on a smile and a shoeshine".*
> Arthur Miller, *Death of a Salesman*

Top People's Shoe Shine

The correct way to clean and shine shoes, courtesy of George Hancock, who shines shoes at Harrods.

TO REMOVE GRIT, MUD AND SALT "Brush shoes off with a hard shoe brush to get all grit out of the welt. Next wash with saddle soap – if the shoes are damp use the saddle soap dry and if the shoes are dry use the saddle soap wet in order to wash off all mud and salt. Capable of clearing horse sweat off tack, saddle soap will remove anything harmful from shoes.

DRYING OUT WET SHOES Don't put shoe trees inside wet shoes as this stops them breathing and keeps the moisture inside. Put paper inside them instead, which will soak up the moisture and allow the shoes to dry. Then apply saddle soap. Never put shoes in a warm place to dry unless you apply saddle soap first.

AN EVERYDAY SHOE SHINE Apply a coat of wax polish with a good brush, neither too small nor so big that it will spray the polish everywhere. Next brush with a soft shoe brush and finally buff up with a well-used yellow duster.

AN ARMY SHINE – SPIT AND POLISH The Americans call this a "spit shine" but you don't spit, obviously. So you take a damp cloth and you work away dipping your cloth into the wax polish and working the polish into the shoe with a circular motion. This is feeding the leather and building up the surface shine. It can take

---

a long time and depends on liberal use of elbow grease. You must keep working the polish in until it has all disappeared, a lot of people give up too soon. When all the polish has gone from the surface buffing up a shine should be easy. Use an old yellow duster – not a new one as that only leaves fluff. A proper spit and polish will give a shine that will last a couple of weeks, all you have to do in the interim is brush the welt but not the top, simply buff that up."

Saving our Soles

Don't wait until shoes are worn right down before taking them to be repaired. Heels wear unevenly, and if you can slide the flat end of a pencil under any part of the edge of your heel it is time they were repaired.

Local specialist shoe repairers, as opposed to while-you-wait heel bars, can offer sound advice and a range of services.

Shoe trees will help to keep shoes in shape between wearings and using a shoe horn will prevent the backs of slip-on style shoes from being trodden down.

Always keep spare laces – shoe laces have a way of snapping when you are about to leave home for an important meeting. . .

No More Blots on the Landscape

There's many a man who moves through life as a testimony to past dinners, old pens and impromptu repairs to his motor car. When your clothes do get stains on them, if you know what to do and act quickly you can often deal with the problem.

Clothes labelled "Dry Clean Only" should really be taken to a good dry cleaners after dry solids have been scraped off gently or liquid spills blotted off with a tissue. Tell the cleaners what has caused the stain so that they can use the correct method of treatment.

Stains on washable materials will be easier to remove if you:

- Deal with them promptly to stop them setting.
- Avoid rubbing as it only pushes a stain further into the fabric.
- Always work from the outside of a stain towards the middle to stop a ring forming.
- Try stain removers on a hidden part of the garment first to make sure it is safe to use on the garment.

HOW TO USE ABSORBENT PADS. . . . Take two absorbent pads of cotton wool, one soaked in solvent and the other held against the stain. Dab the underside with stain remover and the stain will be transferred from the material to the top pad. Turn this round to a clean part and keep working like this until no more staining matter comes through.

To deal with old, dried-in stains, lubricate with glycerine. Apply a mixture of one part glycerine to two parts of water to the stain. Leave this for ten minutes before treating as for fresh stains.

You can treat most stains with a solution of biological detergent and warm water or washing up liquid and warm water. Other useful stain removing agents worth keeping at home are white vinegar, bicarbonate of soda, methylated spirit, a proprietary grease solvent and turpentine.

If you don't want to chance home cures you can always buy one of the many proprietary stain removers, marketed to remove a variety of different stains from chewing gum to tar. Sold at hardware stores, they cost little more than a pint of beer.

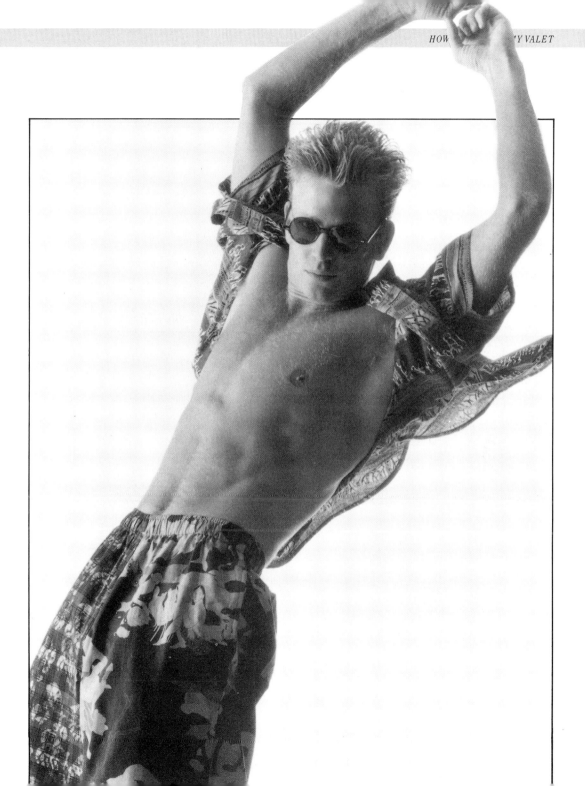

Common stains and traditional cures

A list of the type of stains you may want to deal with and accepted methods of removal. Try them at your own risk, however, as some solvents are toxic, flammable and could affect the colour of a fabric.

ALCOHOL, COFFEE, TEA
Sponge with detergent or washing-up liquid solution and wash as usual. Beer responds well to soaking for a while in solution.

ANTI-PERSPIRANTS
Treat with a paste of bicarbonate of soda and salt, leave on for quarter of an hour. Soak in detergent solution and wash as usual.

OIL
Use proprietary grease solvent and absorbent pad method before washing as usual.

PAINT
Emulsion – Blot off excess, rinse off affected part with cold water and work in neat washing-up liquid. If this does not work ask your dry cleaner for help. Fresh emulsion should wash off, dried stains are very likely permanent.

Gloss – Use turpentine with the absorbent pad method before washing as usual.

PERSPIRATION
Sponge with white vinegar, rinse thoroughly and wash as usual.

RED WINE
Mop up then cover the stain with salt to remove remainder. Sponge with detergent solution, rinse off with cold water and wash as usual as soon as possible.

BALLPOINT PEN AND FELT-TIP
Use methylated spirit with the absorbent pad method before rubbing with soap or a detergent paste and washing as usual.

BLOOD
Soak in well salted cold water, changing salt water repeatedly until it runs clear. Remaining stains can be sponged with detergent or washing-up liquid solution. Then wash in biological powder before it dries.

CHEWING GUM
Rub the gum with an ice cube to harden it, scrape off with a blunt knife and wash as usual. Alternatively use methylated spirit and absorbent pad method before washing.

SHOE POLISH
Lubricate the stain with glycerine then use a propriet-ary grease solvent with the absorbent pad method. Wash as usual.

TAR
Scrape off surplus then use proprietary grease solvent with absorbent pad method, rinse and wash as soon as possible. Alternatively soften with glycerine, work in neat washing-up liquid, rinse with warm water and wash.

Note Do not soak wool, silk, leather or garments with metal fasteners.

LIPSTICK AND MAKE-UP
Treat with proprietary grease solvent and wash in usual way. Alternatively soak up with talc, work in neat washing-up liquid and wash as usual.

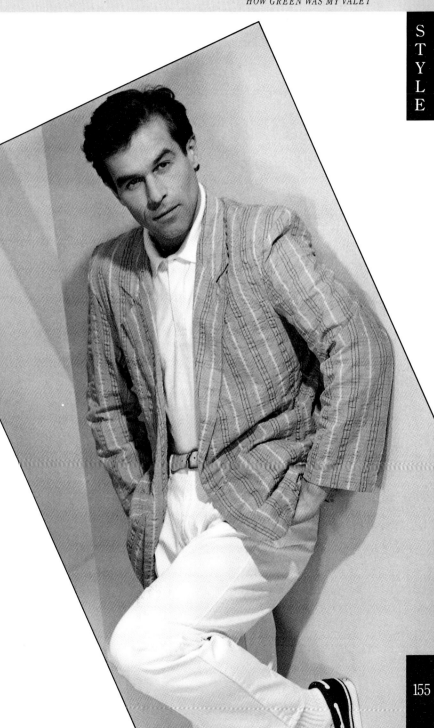

A WASH WITH LABELS

The exotic looking hieroglyphics found on labels in the collars or waistbands and side seams of your clothes are not the latest codes for international spies but care labels, telling you how to clean and care for garments.

BASIC SYMBOLS FOUND ON CARE LABELS

The International Textile Care Labelling Code consists of five symbols:

 for washing (by hand or machine)

 for bleaching

 for tumble drying (after washing)

 for ironing

 for dry cleaning

The symbols should always be presented in the same sequence. They may be found arranged vertically or horizontally.

If any of these symbols has a cross X over it, it means "do not" for that process.

BLEACHING

 Chlorine bleach may be used

 Do not use chlorine bleach

TUMBLE DRYING

 May be tumble dried

 Do not tumble dry

IRONING

The number of dots in the ironing symbol indicate the correct temperature setting – the fewer the dots the cooler the iron setting.

cool   *warm*   *hot*   *do not iron*

DRY CLEANING
May be dry cleaned

The circle may contain letters A, P or F, depending on the requirements or limitations of the article itself. If the circle has a bar beneath it special treatment is required and advice should be sought from a professional dry cleaner.

 Do not dry clean

WASHING INSTRUCTIONS

Care labels giving washing instructions have recently been changed. The changes allow for improvements in modern fabrics, washing machines and detergents. They make it easier to organize mixed washloads.

The introduction of a bar beneath the wash tub means that the washing action should be reduced. A broken bar shows that only the most gentle action is required (usually for fabrics containing wool or silk). The bar replaces the code number used previously. The maximum temperature will be given in the washtub in degrees C and for the time being words may also be added.

WASHING INSTRUCTIONS

OLD	NEW	Examples of Application
		White cotton and linen articles without special finishes
		Cotton, linen or viscose articles without special finishes where colours are fast at 60°C
		(Not used in UK) White nylon and white polyester/cotton mixtures are included in 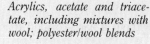
		Nylon; polyester/cotton mixtures; polyester cotton and viscose articles with special finishes; cotton/acrylic mixtures
		Cotton, linen or viscose articles, where colours are fast at 40°C but not at 60°C
		Acrylics, acetate and triacetate, including mixtures with wool; polyester/wool blends
		Wool, wool mixed with other fibres; silk
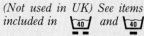		*(Not used in UK) See items included in* 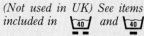 *and*
		(Not applicable in UK)
		Handwash (Do not machine wash)
		Do not wash

THE SIGNIFICANCE OF THE BAR BENEATH THE WASH TUB

No bar ⊔ *normal (maximum) machine action*

Bar ⊔ *reduced (medium) machine action*

Broken bar ⊔ *much reduced (minimum) machine action*

WASH TUBS SHOULD BE LABELLED AS FOLLOWS

⊔ *wash as cotton*

⊔ *wash as synthetics*

⊔ *wash as wool*

In each case a similar phrase, e.g. wash in cotton cycle, wash in cotton programme etc. may be used.

MIXING WASH LOADS

As a general guide you can mix wash labels without a bar provided you wash at the lowest temperature shown.

e.g. ⊔60 *and* ⊔40 *can be washed together at 40°C.*

Likewise, you can mix wash labels with and without a bar provided that, again, you wash at the lowest temperature, BUT you must also reduce the washing action.

e.g. ⊔60 *and* ⊔40 *can be washed together at 40°C at a reduced action.*

Articles with ⊔40 *must be washed as wool at a much reduced action.*

REMEMBER "wash separately" means what it says.

HANDWASH

When a garment is labelled *hand wash only* do not soak for long periods, rub too vigorously, or use very hot water. Rinse thoroughly before drying.

FABRIC CONDITIONERS

Are useful to stop static and clinging. Always use the prescribed amount and mix thoroughly in water. Never use neat on garments.

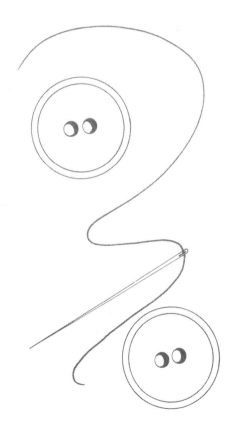

A STITCH IN TIME

Try to sew buttons back on as soon as they come adrift or better still secure ones that are loose before they fall off. Modern shirts usually have machine-stitched buttons and pulling one thread can unravel the lot. If you deal with it promptly you will avoid problems of finding a replacement.

If you have to buy replacements (keeping a card or two at home saves last minute problems), button sizes come in "lignes". Shirt buttons are usually 18 ligne, buttons for jacket fronts from 24–28 ligne and for jacket cuffs 22 ligne. Take your jacket to match up buttons and ask for help in a specialist shop if in doubt.

Use a middle-sized needle from a packet of household needles and buy button thread for jackets and sewing thread for shirts. If your jacket has backing buttons, match them if possible, but a shirt button in a suitable colour will act as a stand in.

Replace four-hole buttons or two-hole buttons with ones that match, not a different variety as this looks tacky. Sew two-hole buttons on with parallel stitches, four-hole buttons can be sewn with parallel bars or with crosses – match existing stitches.

Work with a double thread no longer than the length from your finger tips to your elbow. After the first couple of stitches, pull the button up and hold it about a finger's depth away from the cloth, forming a stalk. After half-a-dozen stitches wind your cotton around the stalk before taking the thread through to the back of the material and securing with several more stitches across the back of the button. This will ensure that fabric does not get torn out. To save frustration check after the first couple of stitches that you've got the button properly positioned.

acknowledgments

The pictures in this book appear by kind permission of:

Aramis; Elizabeth Arden; Giorgio Armani; Associated Press; J. Barbour; Beecham plc; BHS; The Body Shop; Braun; The British Museum; Brylcreem; The Burton Group; C&A; Church & Co; Cossack; Clynol; Crombie of Scotland; De Beers; Denman Brushes; Diamond Information Centre; Christian Dior; Alfred Dunhill; Dunhill; Taylor Ferguson of Glasgow; Joshua Galvin; Gillette; Glemby Editorial; Fringe; 365 Day Hairdressing; Headmaster; Home Laundering Consultative Council; Hornes; Alan International; Innoxa; International Wool Secretariat; Jaeger; Philip Kingsley Trichological Clinic; Klammer Skiwear; Lagerfeld; L'Oreal; Options; Mail Newspapers; Dr M. W. May; Charlie Miller of Edinburgh; Moss Bros; The Museum of London; Nevica; Tommy Nutter; Next For Men; Principles For Men; Austin Reed; Roger & Gallet; Helena Rubenstein; Russell and Bromley; Sabre Knitwear; Vidal Sassoon; Scissors; Selfridges Beauty Playground; Shulton (GB) Ltd; Skin Fitness; Alan Stewart's Rainbow Room; Tabac; The Tie Rack; Truefitt & Hill; Van Heusen; Viennaline; Stephen Way; Wella; Wilkinson Sword Ltd; Young's Formal Wear; Yves Saint Laurent.

The editor and authors wish to thank the following for their invaluable help in preparing this book:

Alan International; Aramis; Arlington Socks; Laraine Ashton Model Agency; The Associaton of Optical Practitioners; Nina Bacon; J. Barbour; The Bear Inn, Oxford; Bic; BHS; Boots; Anita Roddick of The Body Shop; Braun; The British Clothing Centre; The British Clothing Industry Association; The British Shoe Corporation; The British Man Made Fibres Federation; The British Red Cross Society; The Burton Group; C&A; Charles of the Ritz; Church and Co; Clinique; Clynol; Sharon Dale; 365 Day Hairdressing; Suzanne Barton of Dickens and Jones; Dollond and Aitchison; Colin Cairns of Dunn and Co; Du Pont; Joshua Galvin; Gillette UK Ltd; Harrods; The Institute of Electrolysis; The Ivy Shop, Richmond; Harrods; Hacketts; Hermès; Hoechst; Home Laundering Consultative Council; Judy James; G. B. Kent and Sons; Glenn Lyons of the Philip Kingsley Trichological Clinic; Knickerbox; Lever Bros; Lillywhites; Leonard of Mayfair International; Marks & Spencer; Menswear Association of Great Britain; Millett's; Jeff Marsh of The Museum of London; Moss Bros; Mark Nicholas; Nike; Tommy Nutter; Optical Information Council; Optyl; Pentagram Designs Ltd; Philips; John Jelieneck of Principles for Men; Remington; The Ritz; The Royal Navy; Sabre; Elliott Grant of Vidal Sassoon; Jane Pickering of Seeber Consumer Pharmaceuticals; Selfridges Beauty Playground; Silhouette Ltd; Sketchley's Ltd; John Field of Skin Fitness; Slimmer Menswear; Irene Shuman of Snip and Sew; Mr Spooner of Peterborough; The Sock Shop; Steiner Products Ltd; Textile Market Studies; The Tie Rack; Tootal; Turnbull and Asser; Truefitt & Hill; George F. Trumper; Van Heusen; Viyella Menswear; Wilkinson Sword Ltd.

index